P9-DWS-602

# THE GOOD LIVING GUIDE TO

# NATURAL AND HERBAL REMEDIES

SIMPLE SALVES, TEAS, TINCTURES, AND MORE

# KATOLEN YARDLEY, MNIMH

MEMBER OF THE NATIONAL INSTITUTE OF MEDICAL HERBALISTS

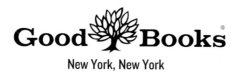
Good Books

New York, New York

Good Books books may be purchased in bulk at special discounts for sales promotion, corporate gifts, fund-raising, or educational purposes. Special editions can also be created to specifications. For details, contact the Special Sales Department, Good Books, 307 West 36th Street, 11th Floor, New York, NY 10018 or info@skyhorsepublishing.com.

Good Books is an imprint of Skyhorse Publishing, Inc.®, a Delaware corporation.

Visit our website at www.goodbooks.com.

10 9 8 7 6 5 4 3 2 1

Library of Congress Cataloging-in-Publication Data is available on file.

Cover design by Jenny Zemanek

Print ISBN: 978-1-68099-157-4
Ebook ISBN: 978-1-68099-158-1

Printed in China

# TABLE OF CONTENTS

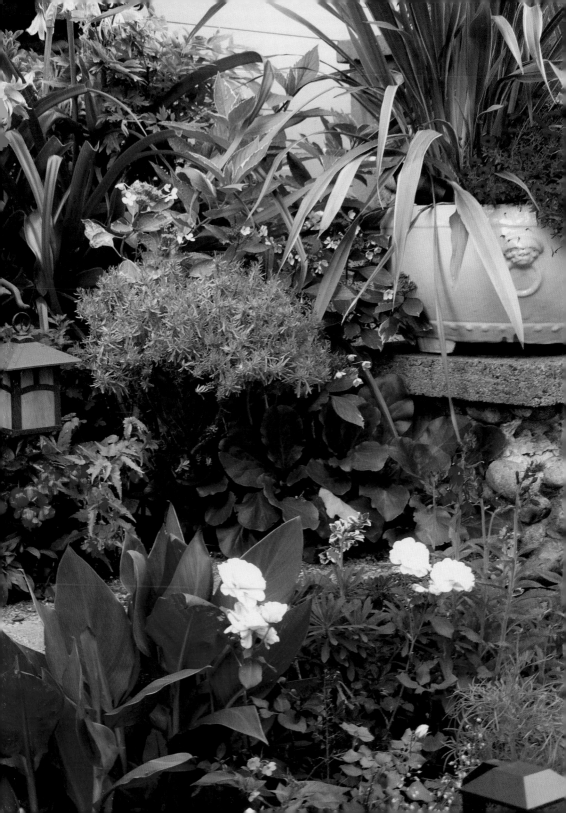

# Acknowledgments

Confirming my belief that everything occurs for a higher reason, the opportunity to write this book presented itself and developed at the perfect time. Thank you to the publisher, Abigail, and Jennifer Browne for the synchronistic unfoldments leading up to this book.

Lluis Amoros, this book is for you on the day of Sant Jordi, *el día del libro y de la rosa*. To my dear ones Rod Frew and Marcia Clingman: for your willingness to stay present and explore the unknown. To my dear friends, especially Rob Fisher and Sean Cook, for the opportunity for heartfelt sharing and moments of connection: your presence has been a consistent encouragement. To all my clients who have reciprocated stories, dreams, laughter, and fears—your presence has enriched this journey called life. Thank you for continuing to teach me and for reminding me of the importance of connection.

Thank you to my mentors, teachers, and fellow herbalists— both inspirations in their own ways—Chanchal Cabrera, FNIMH, and herbalist Rowan Hamilton, for fueling my mind's need for philosophical contemplation and possibility. Christopher Hedley, with whom I apprenticed while studying in the UK, taught me the necessity of getting back in touch with nature and plants. When I was ill while studying abroad, he entered his kitchen and blended a valuable bronchitis syrup for me at a moment's notice, thereby instilling the importance of accessible medicine for everyone.

## Disclaimer

The information contained within this book is not intended to diagnose, treat, cure, or prevent any disease, and it is not in any way a substitute for professional advice. If you have an ongoing medical condition, it is essential to consult your health-care provider before embarking on any self-treatment. Before implementing any of this information, each individual is responsible for weighing the risks and benefits. He or she may want to seek medical advice first and be monitored periodically by a doctor or health-care provider while employing these practices. It is the responsibility of the health-care provider, relying on the unique health history of each individual, to determine the correct dosage and treatment for any particular person. This information is for educational purposes only and does not convey or warrant, either expressly or implied, any guaranteed outcomes, promises, or benefits from this protocol. When harvesting wild plants, it is imperative that you identify the species correctly. Neither the publisher nor the author is responsible for any omissions or errors of any kind; nor do they assume any liability for injury and/or damage to persons or property arising from this publication. As new research and clinical experience are revealed, modifications with treatment protocols may be necessary. It is the responsibility of the reader to check the most up-to-date information regarding dosage, contraindications, and duration of use.

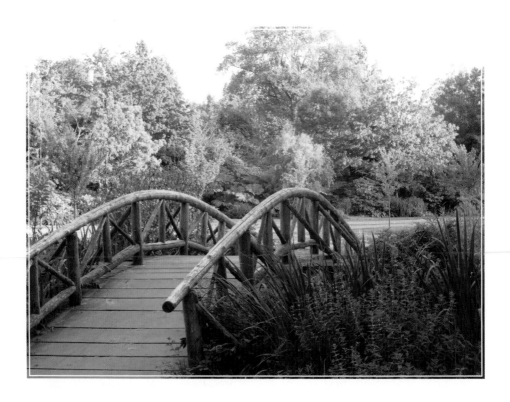

# Introduction

My passion for herbal medicine has spanned over twenty years, including incredible visits to the jungle to learn about exotic medicinal plants, adventures in third-world countries to observe different cultural and traditional health-care and spiritual practices, and climbing local mountains to discover medicinal plants growing in my own backyard. In private practice, my area of expertise focuses on digestive health, skin conditions, and female reproductive health issues; in addition, for close to twenty years, I have taught herbal medicine-making techniques in schools and to the general public. I have been in private practice as a medical herbalist since 1999, and both my clients and the plants I use continue to be my teachers.

Accessible and environmentally-friendly practices provide sustainability for our health and the planet. If a vision for a cleaner future exists for our planet, and if there is wisdom for improved ways of living life, then it is our responsibility to be a part of that momentum. A humble approach is to focus on the results we wish to see. For any change to occur in industrial practices and the contamination of our planet with industrial waste, we need to first recognize the intrinsic value of Mother Earth, her plants, and all species on this planet. Herbal medicine can be considered preventive medicine providing accessible medicine for many; it holds value through its ability to lower costs for the overburdened health-care system and for its contribution toward the ongoing stability of the planet. It offers us tools to maintain the fragile balance of our ecosystem and to remember our connection to all life on this planet. If herbs are used in a green, renewable fashion, then plant medicine can help ensure a viable future for the next generations.

I am writing this book as an herbalist, and my angle is to share the various ways and possibilities to incorporate herbal medicines into our daily lifestyle—as food when available, as medicine when appropriate, and as a method and reminder of the accessibility and importance of sustainable practices for the health of our planet. It is my preference to use plant medicine and become familiar with plants prior to recommending them to clients. With frequency of use, confidence increases and misconceptions and hesitations diminish.

This book provides health and home remedies. It contains insights on how we heal, including an introduction to common herbs and foods that can be utilized for what ails us. There are numerous recipes for food, first aid, family health issues, and body care contained within these pages.

The use of plants for healing our ills is the oldest form of therapy—plants offer vast capacities in terms of our healing and play a vital role in our remembering. Most importantly, this book is about connection. It is a tool to remind us of our lost connection with nature, which supplies both our food and medicine, and the importance of caring for Mother Earth which provides life on our planet.

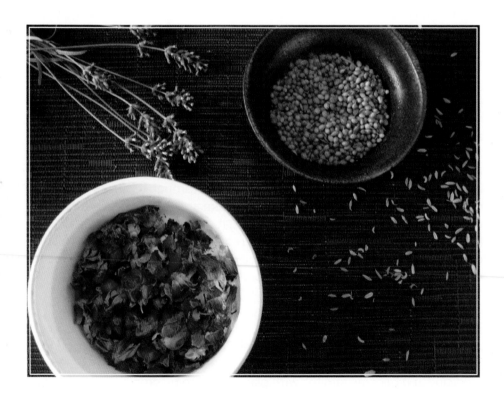

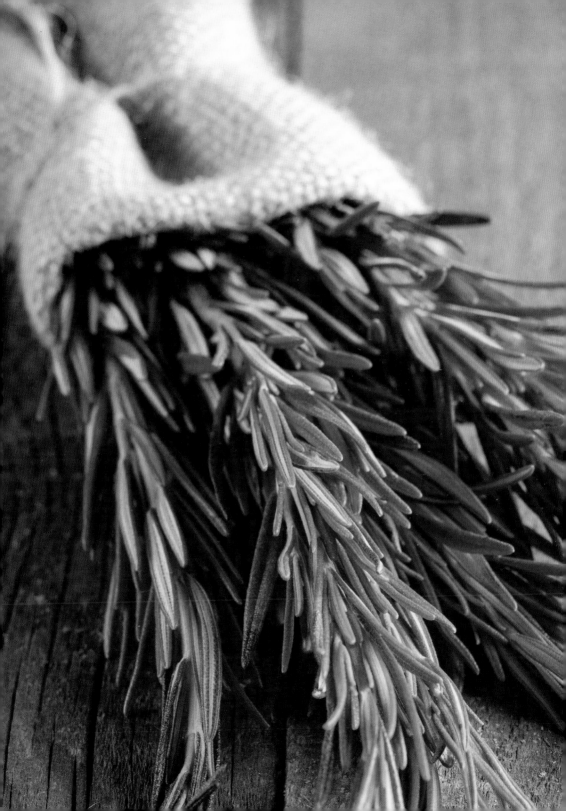

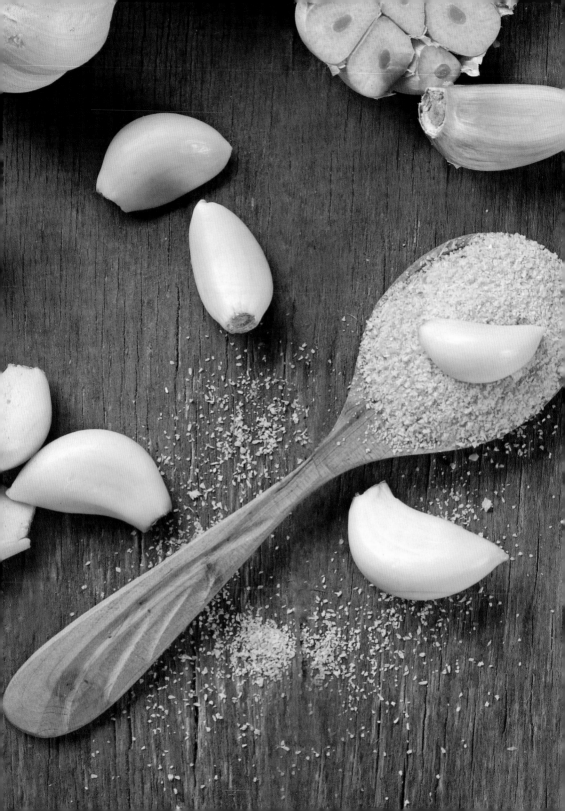

# BACKGROUND AND GETTING STARTED

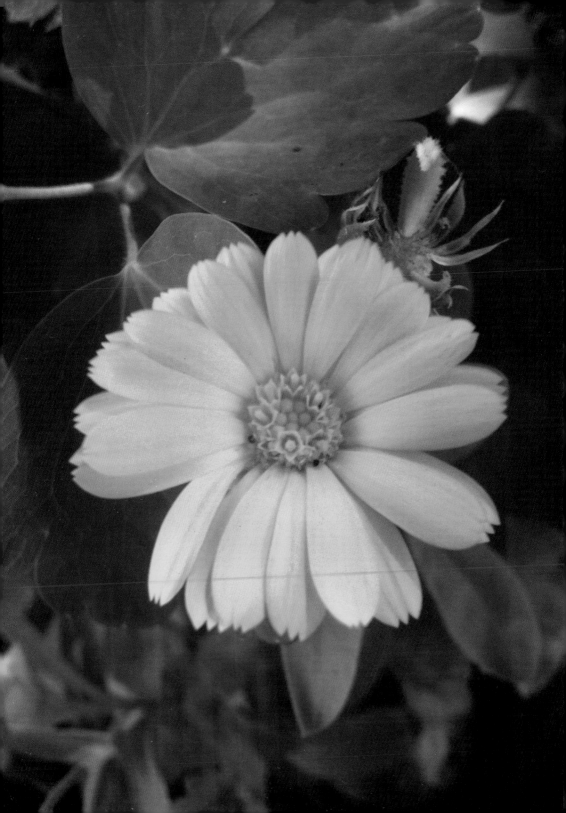

# A Journey of Evolution: Plant and Human Relations

All living things on this planet depend on plant life to survive. Just like humans, plants are live beings. They take in our carbon dioxide and convert it to oxygen through photosynthesis. They are an essential part of our breathing cycle as they clean the air we breathe. The exchange of breath is our connection to the natural world and to source energy (call it God, spirit, a higher power, Gaia, the divine). Being alive and interacting with the environment just like human beings, plants are our allies, provided by Mother Nature to nourish and assist with what ails us.

Plants take in nourishment from the sun and soil, just as humans ingest foods provided by nutrient-rich soil. The nutrients within plants assist in our healing. Plants contain chemical constituents that provide natural protection from insects (nature's insecticides), viruses, and bacteria. Some examples of these natural pesticides and insecticides include anthocyanins, sulforaphane, and volatile oils. Plants release agents into the air to ensure protection from insects. In doing so, these volatile oils have the ability to affect communication with other plants in the same area, warning of an impending danger. Many of these antioxidant, nutrient-rich compounds "are therapeutic in the treatment of many diseases including heart disease, cancer, diabetes, arthritis, lupus, neurological disorders, and fibromyalgia"[1] and offer antimicrobial effects and immune activity against pathogens in our own bodies. Essential oils also exhibit broad agricultural possibility. For example, natural insecticides provide more effective fumigant activity for grain protection than some chemical pesticides without the associated risks of synthetic insecticides.[2]

# Plants as Teachers

Nature certainly provides tools for us to awaken and to heal. Plants "give out" more than they take in. This very contemplation could give pause for reflection on the extent of our own consumerism. Plants can be viewed as our teachers.

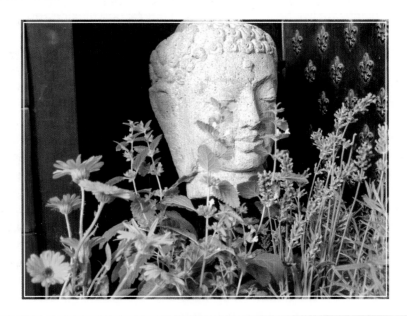

Observing a plant's life cycle teaches us valuable life lessons. The simple act of planting a seed and waiting for it to germinate teaches us patience. The strongest forces are often unseen, with much force beneath the surface (consider electricity or radio waves, for example). The cultivation of faith exists when no results are visible, yet unseen forces are building according to the predominant focus and in line with the desired outcome. Planting a seed teaches us perseverance in times when faith is all there is.

Nature provides a path back to harmonious connection: fellowship with our community and a link to our higher selves. Nature can be a refuge, restoring safety and trust. Consider it a neural network reset button for those who have experienced emotional trauma (PTSD) and are daily reliving pain, anxiety, and suffering. Like the healing capacities of a loving, furry, four-legged friend, nature provides the quiet calm so needed to reset a triggered nervous system. It shows us a solid path to realign in harmony with all our relations and create associations more in line with the flow of Mother Earth. Although somewhat humorous-sounding, even so-called "tree hugging" has now been validated by the scientific community. In the book *Blinded by Science*, Matthew Silverstone speaks of nature's ability to facilitate an improved sense of wellbeing, or "relief by communing with trees." First Nations' philosophies have long revered trees as being a sacred part of community. They view trees as one of Mother Nature's healers, able to absorb negative energy. Silverstone seconds this view by suggesting that the subtle vibration or vital life force of trees, deeply rooted with earth energy, facilitates the transformation of energy into one of peace-filled unity.

Plants have personalities. As with people, some plants are mild, gentle, and nourishing while others are strong, potent herbs that demand our respect for safe use. Through sacred ceremony, plant-spirit medicines are gifted with louder voices for more direct communication and reconnection with plant-realm relationships, facilitating emotional healing and well-being and reminding us that we are all connected. What we do to the earth, we do to ourselves. Learning to listen to the subtle teachings of plants involves listening more with our hearts and less with our ears in order to receive the gifts our green friends can offer.

We inherit the earth. How do we responsibly care for the gift we have been given?

# Is a Plant a Food or Is It Considered a Medicine?

Many foods from other cultures (and also plants grown in our own gardens) have been held in high regard for their healing qualities, known as nutrient-rich superfoods and sometimes called "herbal medicine." Modern research is confirming the health benefits of flavonoid and antioxidant-rich fruit and cruciferous vegetables for immune health, as foods that help to reduce inflammation, prevent cancer, and offer protection from the development of chronic diseases.

The shift from seeing food as essential nourishment to ingesting herbs as medicine is subtle. Many common foods ingested daily in both ethnic cultures and our own diets are a form of herbal medicine. What has been lost is the knowledge and wisdom of how to apply these plants, our foods, as effective medicine. Utilizing the medicines that Mother Earth provides as healing tools may be one of the long roads back to finding more harmony and vibrant health.

In Asia, gobo is a common root vegetable (herbalists know this parsnip-like root as burdock). Burdock is a nutritive food and an alterative or "blood cleanser" for cellular detoxification. It is effective for removal of uric acid buildup from the joints. Maca is a turnip and food staple for the indigenous populations in the Andes of Peru. While the foods grown in various climates of other continents are valuable, there is much to be said for the superfoods in our own backyards. Many of our common plants, even weeds, have yet to be fully appreciated. In my opinion, broccoli, parsley, and dandelion are some of our own local super plants. Bitter dandelion greens are not only a chef's delight but also herbal medicines. Similarly, the cardiovascular protective properties of garlic have been studied, yet is it not a food? Like dandelion, it is the same plant, just a different paradigm and point of comparison.

I often reflect on our current health paradigm and observe the focus on studying illness rather than researching habits of health and optimal well-being. I support practices that focus on sustainability, nutrient-rich soils, high-nutrient foods, and activities that contribute to enhanced healing, harmony, and a community of peace and joy for all rather than practices that fuel disease, create separation, and deplete our natural resources. Shouldn't accessibility to quality, nutrient-rich, healing foods be the bottom line? Why not develop new ways of researching, utilizing, and preserving nature's healers rather than depleting natural resources?

Foods found in our kitchens such as cabbage, carrots, and onions are very nutritious and—when used with healing wisdom—also have medicinal properties. Flavonoid-rich berries like blueberries, blackberries, and raspberries contain anti-inflammatory properties. Inflammation is now considered one of the contributing causes of chronic degenerative disease. Also, local herbs such as rose hips, nettles, and chickweed are all valuable foods that contain unique healing properties.

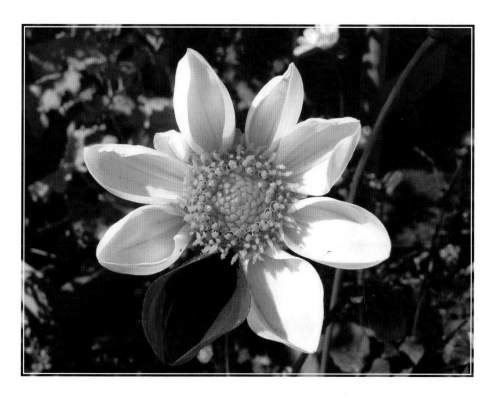

# Herbal Medicine Worldwide

Herbal medicine is still the primary form of medicine used worldwide. Not only is it used by up to 80 percent of the population in Asia and Africa, but around 25 percent of modern pharmaceutical drugs, including aspirin, digitalis, morphine, taxol, and quinine, have been derived from plants. In fact, over seven thousand chemical compounds currently used in modern drug manufacturing are directly sourced from plants.[3,4,5]

It is a known fact that "pharmaceuticals are both an unaffordable and unobtainable option to many; with over half of the world's population living on less than $2 per day—herbal medicines, in contrast, can be grown from organic seeds or sustainably gathered from nature."[6,7] Plants are renewable resources (when replanted and sustainably harvested) and do not contribute to environmental pollution produced by pharmaceuticals; they remain the people's medicine—both affordable and accessible and used by many cultures as the first medicinal option.

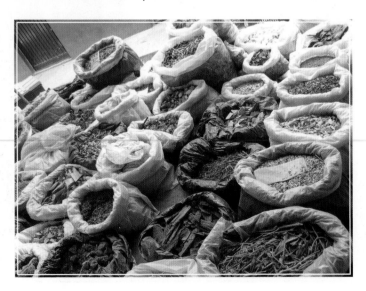

## Food for Thought

Medicines are valuable in the right circumstances; however, it is important to keep in mind the vested interests behind the marketing of any packaged product. Consider for a moment the profits obtained by Big Pharma patenting isolated chemicals derived from what nature herself provides. According to the World Health Organization, "the global pharmaceuticals market is worth $300 billion a year, a figure expected to rise to $400 billion within three years. The ten largest drug companies control over one-third of this market, several with sales of more than $10 billion a year and profit margins of about 30%."[8] To put this in perspective, when asked what it would cost to eliminate world hunger, the United Nations estimated only 30 billion per year![9] Big Pharma is capitalism at its best . . . and worst. The return to using plant medicine puts health care back in the hands of the people and away from big business.

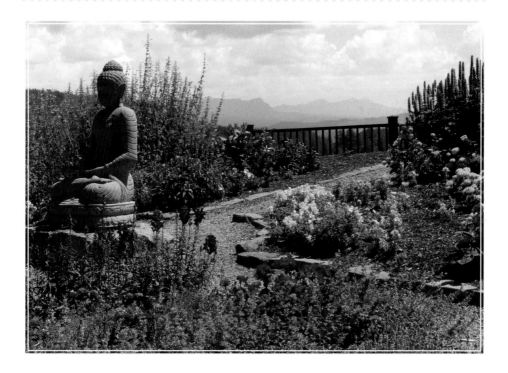

# Possibilities for Plants in Your Life

Since 1998, I have had the privilege of providing herbal, nutritional, and holistic wellness solutions on an "Ask an Expert" news segment for a long-running, nationally syndicated news program. As their guest medical herbalist, I have answered viewers' questions on a range of chronic health issues, providing a starting place for health enhancement and focusing their attention on some possible underlying issues and root causes of disease. Through this medium I have witnessed a demand for preventive tools, herbal options for improved care and observed how nutritional choices play a large role in our overall health.

With nearly two decades of experience serving thousands of clients in private practice, I have observed a correlation that what we put in, on, and around our bodies can wreak havoc on our endocrine, immune, digestive, and reproductive systems, causing many forms of disease. I have also witnessed many individuals transform their health issues and maintain improvements in disease over long periods of time by addressing their lifestyle and nutrition, and by supporting their bodies with herbal medicine.

When people consume foods deficient in proper nutrients or when our bodies absorb the unhealthy substances found in products heavily laden with artificial chemicals, pesticides, and environmental toxins (such as processed foods), our biological environment is altered, making it challenging to sustain optimal vibrant health.

I am acutely aware of the symbiotic relationship humans have with Mother Earth and the urgency of recognizing and remembering her value as we, and all of our living allies, coexist on her planet.

Nature can provide for our needs. It has been said that healing for all ailments exists on this planet; however, a vast number of the Earth's plant populations exist in jungles that are either yet to be discovered or soon to be destroyed. Thus, now is the time to bring awareness to our responsibility for sustaining this interdependent relationship, to recognize the plants that Mother Nature provides for our health. Positive change occurs when we focus on the intended outcome and take appropriate action.

When used properly, herbal medicines are powerful healing agents. Many common foods and local weeds are also valuable medicines. Herbs can be considered the first option of treatment for common health issues and body care.

If plant medicine is considered a valued resource, then future generations will more likely preserve what they know and care for. Children who are taught the importance of a healthy earth and educated to understand both the impact of pollution and the importance of health maintenance may consider solutions for a cleaner world. By incorporating natural remedies and body care items into everyday use, you can take advantage of their numerous benefits while minimizing any adverse impact on the environment.

*"What is a weed? A plant whose virtues have never been discovered." —Ralph Waldo Emerson*

People are curious about using plants to take charge of their health but often don't know where to start.

- "How can I use plants in new ways for my health?"
- "What should I do to ensure the desired outcome and safety when using herbal medicines?"
- "Which choices are the most environmentally friendly?"
- "Where do I begin?"

Begin right where you are! Learn about the medicinal properties of items you already have in your spice cupboard, fridge, and garden—both herbs and common foods. Build your confidence by learning the medicinal properties and applications of plants with which you are already familiar.

Consider plants as both a source of nourishment and healing. Just as high-octane gasoline can make your car operate better, nutrient-dense foods fuel a high-performance body. Similarly, what we put in and on our body has an impact on its performance. However, unlike a car, your body has an extraordinary capacity for regeneration.

Therefore, the first and perhaps most important aspect to a vital, strong body is to ensure you are choosing the best fuel. Our choice of nourishment is a basic starting point; if a food does not come directly from the soil or grow from a tree in its whole form, then it should not be eaten on a regular basis.

The second step is to build good habits through awareness that what we put in and on our body will impact our health. As creatures of habit, we often resort to what is most familiar. For example, if you were raised in a family that used aspirin regularly to ease the body's expression of pain and discomfort, then this may be your default choice, without much hesitation or thought about the long-term consequences to your digestive system. Similarly, the actions we observe in our families become models of behavior that we easily adopt for ourselves. So, there is always value in reflecting on our habits and making conscious choices for the behavior in our families. Health-filled habits will benefit everyone long-term. Incorporating plant medicines into daily routines offers something for everyone. Recipes are fun to make, and if you can involve children, you will create a learning environment (an educational opportunity to learn about the body and how it functions) that benefits the whole family.

Herbs can be used for almost any ailment for which one might visit the doctor. Herbal medicines also offer effective alternatives to common first aid; they can address acute health issues by tending to a cut or scrape with a disinfectant or a poultice for pulling out a sliver or soothing a sore throat. Creating an herbal first aid kit is a great place to begin when using herbs regularly. Herbs can offer support for more long-term complaints such as allergies, hives, and indigestion. Plants can activate our bodies' self-healing capacities by providing nourishment and vitamin support, encouraging elimination of waste and toxins, and by strengthening and supporting organ systems for improved health. Plants can also be used to create natural cosmetics and non-toxic body care and home cleaning products. These plant-based products are less toxic for the environment than many consumer products currently on the market.

Although valuable in their own right, "heavy hitters" such as prescription drugs, medical interventions, and surgery, can be reserved as the very last option after lifestyle modifications have been addressed and all natural alternatives have been exhausted.

When we reserve stronger treatments only for those ailments and emergencies that may not be resolved competely with natural remedies, everyone benefits: family health care is effectively addressed at a lower cost, the burden on the health-care system is lifted, and people can limit the potential side effects of pharmaceuticals. Moreover, the incidence of iatrogenic disease, (complications arising from allopathic or mainstream medical pharmaceutical treatments) is reduced. For example, aspirin is linked to gastric bleeding, antihistamines in some circumstances can actually cause hives,[10] and the birth control pill has been linked to side effects that include an increase in LDL cholesterol, decreased libido, breast pain, increased risk of estrogen-dependent breast cancers,[11,12,13] depression,[14] blood clots,[15] candidia yeast infections,[16,17] and an increased risk of cervical cancers.[18]

Healing plants can be discovered just outside your doorstep. You may find medicinal plants growing around the neighborhood, mingling in grass, hanging out along roadways, in parks, and flourishing in gardens. Many of the so-called weeds can have medicinal properties. Sadly, as these plants have likely come in contact with anti-weed sprays, car fumes, and other toxins, I am not suggesting that you harvest them. But, if you look closely, you will be able to identify and appreciate the plants that are choosing to comingle around your home. Medicinal plants needed for common ailments can often be found growing close by.

# HARVESTING MEDICINES

If you choose to harvest plants from nature, it is critical to correctly identify each species. Ideally, "wild crafting" involves sustainable and respectful harvesting practices to ensure that the plants continue to propagate and provide medicine in the future. Take only what you need. Herbs selected should grow at least forty feet from any roadway or other area of possible pollution, spray, or contamination. Harvest healthy plants only, in the correct season for the needed plant part. Ensure that there are enough plants left to guarantee pollination and reseeding for the future. Respectfully offer a gesture of gratitude, a prayer, or an offering of thanks to Mother Earth for the medicine you are harvesting.

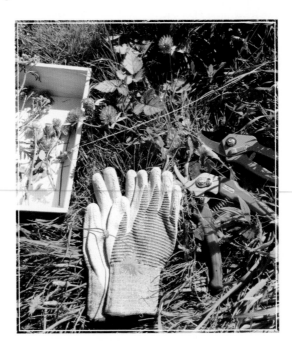

# Essential Requirements for Optimal Health

Plants contain vitamins and minerals that are essential to maintaining the body's daily functioning. Many nutrients are either catalysts, cofactors, or make up enzymes that are involved in maintaining homeostasis. Optimal health can be maintained by ensuring some key requirements:

1. A Strong Connection to Spirit—Perhaps our time on this earth is about strengthening our connection to spirit, every adventure and unexpected turn an opportunity to connect more deeply with the divine.

2. Our Emotional Outlook—Is our cup half empty or half full? The lens through which we view the world (stories we tell ourselves) and our expectations of a positive outcome have an impact on our health. Like a ship's anchor secured to one spot, unresolved emotions of pain, doubt, fear, and anger can be like a brake hindering improved states of health. The release of our grievances and stories of the past is necessary to move forward with the expectation of good things in our future.

3. Adequate Hydration—Life on this planet would cease to exist without clean drinking water. Water bathes our cells by hydrating and diluting toxins for removal. No, coffee does not suffice! Even though it is a liquid, coffee is largely a diuretic and a stimulant, both of which lead to dehydration and an overstimulation of sensitive organs.

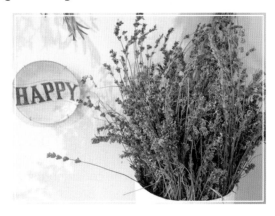

> "Water is fluid, soft, and yielding. But water will wear away rock, which is rigid and cannot yield. As a rule, whatever is fluid, soft, and yielding will overcome whatever is rigid and hard. This is another paradox: what is soft is strong." – Lao Tzu

4. Movement, Movement, Movement!—Flow of the body teaches us to release instead of holding tight to our experiences in life. Observe a willow tree in the breeze, flowing in the breath of life. The branch is not brittle, but instead flexes and bends with the wind. Nature teaches us about flexibility and releasing resistance. All forms of movement (stretching and elongating the body, walking, swimming, and using whole-body vibration machines) are essential for removing waste material from the body and reducing congestion. Refer to the section on the lymphatic system on page 240 for more background.

5. Fresh Clean Air—All too often, we do not realize what we are missing until it is taken away. Much could be said about the importance of fresh air and taking in the invigorating vital energy of Mother Earth. (Refer to Vital Energy Page 27 for more information.) In cities with high air pollution, afflictions like asthma, infections, and breathing difficulties are a common occurrence. We require clean air for our health.

6. Conscious Breath—Breathe into your abdomen using deep, rhythmic belly breaths. Too many of us are "surface breathers," meaning that our inhalation of fresh air is so shallow it is not even apparent, let alone efficient. Deep belly breathing calms the central nervous system instantaneously. The breath assists in strengthening the connection of our mind to our body.

Bring your attention to your breath. In . . . and out. Notice your belly filling with air, and exhale. Stay completely present. Attune, consciously sending the breath deep into your belly then fill up the lungs. Feel the expansiveness. Experience the pause, and witness the slowing down of the body. There is nothing more to do. Breathing consciously takes one out of the looping thoughts and anxiety of the mind. It is the breath that helps get us out of the cycling chatter in our mind and allows us to be more present in our bodies.

What is this thing called Breath? One cannot see the breath unless outside in the frosty cold, yet invisible forces are often the most powerful. Breath is life. It can also be considered a connection to spirit, to *life*, and is shared by all living things. Breath is also synonymous with the vital chi energy that exists in all living things.

## Our Life is Dependent Upon Our Breath.

"Prana" is a Sanskrit term that translates as life-giving force or absolute energy.[19] Though virtually unseen, it is felt as active life energy, a current of electricity throughout the body. Hindu philosophy, as seen in the practice of yoga, speaks of Breath as the fundamental connection between spirit and all things. It is the energy in all living things, an inner vitality, a spark or "life force" that is activated at our first moment of breath and leaves when we transition. This ultimate energy is vital to our existence. Air is Mother Nature's breath, *life* expanding into the world. It is an extension of the spirit of the Creator or cosmic energy and our connection to all things. Our vitality is dependent on our tuning in to this universal life energy.

All higher forms of life utilize breath. Plants function in a symbiotic relationship with us, and we are dependent upon them for the exchange of oxygen and carbon dioxide. Plants, like humans, are alive, contain a vital life force, and assist the body's return to a balanced state. Like plants, our energy field interacts with other living things.

Rhythmic breathing has therapeutic benefit as well. Its practice leads us away from fear and worry and draws us into alignment with the harmonious vibration of nature. Through supporting the energy flow, or prana, vital life force is strengthened. This can be used to invigorate any organ through focusing the breath and consciously directing it to certain areas of the body for healing.

Wilhelm Reich and Freud studied and spoke of this very energy that is present in all living things, which is said to contain the energy of the universe. Delving deeper into this concept, all matter contains an electrical, magnetic field that pulses at a certain frequency and is reactivated by our breathing. In essence, we are taking in the breath of the universe. A form of electrical activity that enables healing, our vital life force flows through chakras or meridians and around us in a broad field called the auric field. There are also energies that can disrupt the flow of life force, including chemicals, preservatives, x-rays, microwave frequencies, and certain types of ionizing electromagnetic frequencies.

To demonstrate this point, many experiments from modern research are confirming that homeostasis[20] and body healing can be facilitated through stimulation of the body's bioelectric fields. Modern research is investigating how pulsing electromagnetic fields help nerve regeneration in rats,[21,22] and static magnetic fields help speed up rates of healing in animals.[23,24]

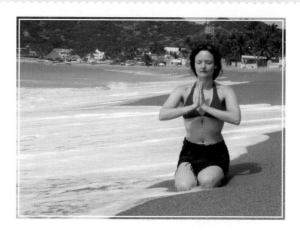

### Instant Calm Practice

Light a candle and place your attention on the flickering flame. Focus on your breath. Breathe in for a count of four, hold for a count of four, breathe out for a count of six, and hold for a count of six. Repeat.

The exhalation is considered by yoga master BK Iyengar as "a sacred act of surrender" that soothes your nervous system, releases the hold of negative emotions, and quiets the mind.

7. Optimal Fuel—There is a fine line between food as medicine and food for nourishment. In fact, are they not the same thing? Plants and humans have shared a long coexistence on this planet, but one hindrance to our health is the growing number of food-like products devoid of naturally-occurring nutrients.

8. Health of the Microbiome and Optimal Functioning of the Digestive Tract—The symbiotic relationship that makes up our inner world, our digestion, is one entry point for foreign agents. Responsible for overseeing the assimilation, absorption, and distribution of nutrients, the function of the digestive tract is so crucial for our health, it is believed that the health of the entire body begins with efficient digestion. Typically, the digestive tract is impermeable and highly selective as to what leaves the intestines and enters the bloodstream. However, leaky gut or increased intestinal permeability (due to overuse of antibiotics, genetically modified ingredients, sugar, pesticides, chemical additives and an assortment of other reasons) is one contributing factor to allergies, food sensitivities, immune system dysfunction, systemic inflammation and chronic degenerative health conditions. We are just beginning to see the cumulative impact of the variety of these assaults on our immune and digestive systems. The digestive system is the eyes and ears of the immune system, with 70 percent of the entire immune system residing in the mucous membranes of the digestive tract.[25,26]

These simple yet fundamental guidelines are key indicators and such essential benchmarks for optimal peak health that I often begin my teaching with these reminders. We are connected to the world which nourishes us and without balance, and connection to our source, disease can develop.

Factors known to contribute to poor health include:
- Alcohol
- Chemical-laden cigarettes
- Sugar
- Food-like-products (full of artificial coloring, additives, preservatives, pesticides, or genetically modified seed stock)
- Leaky gut syndrome
- Stress and anxiety

# Health Imbalances

The simplest understanding of disease in the body results from blockages in the normal flow of vital energy and an interruption of homeostasis through a variety of means. As health is unique to each of us, the cause of disease also varies. Restoring health should ideally focus on the unique history of each person, not only symptomatic treatment. Considering the health of the whole person involves looking at lifestyle, past medical history, emotions, and diet. It also involves considering the impact of cumulative environmental contaminants.[27]

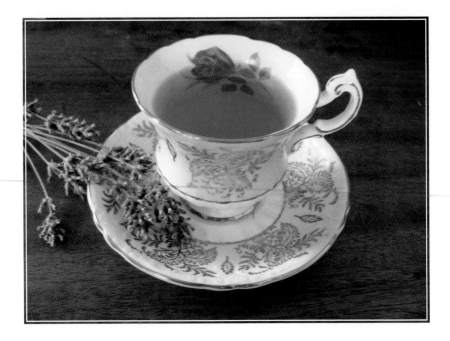

# How We Heal

All improvement in health and healing in the body, regardless the type of medicine or practitioner, is a result of activating the inner vital life force and returning body functions to homeostasis (normal range). Herbal medicine can be used to stimulate this self-healing process by enhancing the body's life force, improving stamina and vitality to encourage improved health. Herbs may support specific organ systems, aid the organs in detoxification, and provide nourishment, but the body itself is the healer.

Any improvement in healing often occurs in a step-like manner; at no point should reaching a plateau be disconcerting. Rest, or a period of no visible activity, is essential to harnessing the vital energies needed to over-throw current states. The strongest stitch in sewing is the backstitch, which takes two steps forward and then one step back. This is a useful analogy for healing. The most crucial healing time is *rest*, the time during the pause.

There is a moment when vital force gains momentum to overcome the current conditions and move into the next step of improved health. If we push our body when it should be at rest, we risk wearing down its natural defenses instead of supporting homeostatic processes.

*"Natural forces within us are the true healers of disease."*
—Hippocrates

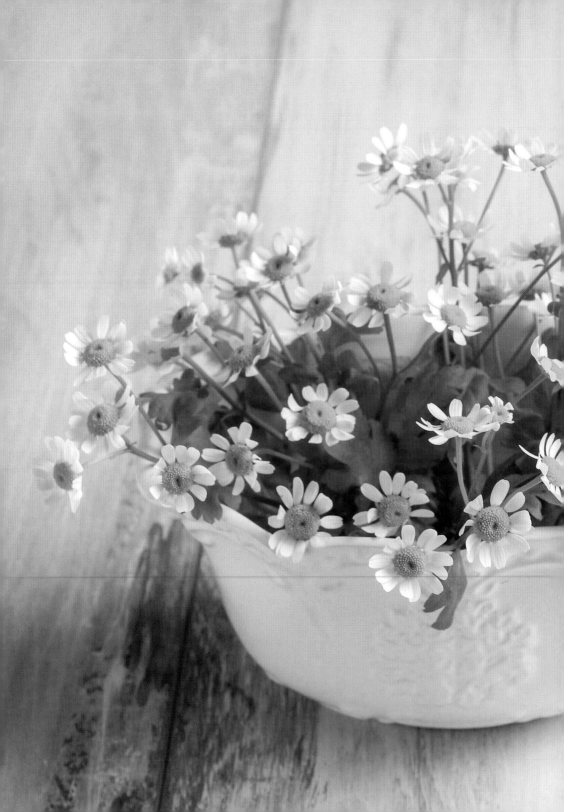

# THE HERBS: BACKGROUND AND USES

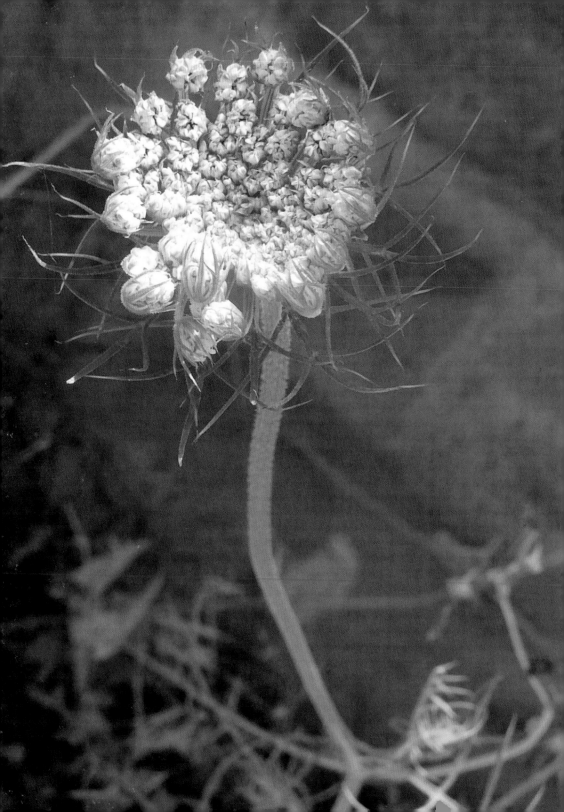

# Mastering Herbal Terminology

## Categorization of Plants

Herbs like antimicrobials, vulneraries, carminatives, and bitters can be understood and categorized according to their main actions in the body. There are a multitude of plants that fit into each category. Dive into embracing the new terminology! Familiarize yourself with plant actions and medical terminology as part of understanding how herbs work. Herbs can be selected to fit the presentations of the client or the desired outcome of a blend. In addition, herbs are categorized by the following considerations:

### For the Love of Latin

Learning the Latin names of plants will expand your skills from that of a local plant lover, where certain "common names" of plants are used, to worldwide access regardless of country or language. No matter where you are in the world, if you know the botanical name of the plant, you will be able to find the very herb you are looking for. Latin names (using both the genus and species name) are the universal language or formal botanical language for plant identification. When writing Latin, the genus name is always capitalized and the species name is lower case: *Stellaria media*. When you encounter the abbreviation "spp.," this indicates several species that may be used interchangeably.

- **Tonic herbs, which build and strengthen the whole body or a specific organ system, are often considered foods in other cultures.** They are nourishing and act as foods, containing high amounts of nutrients required to rebuild and strengthen overall body health. These herbs have been called "simples" because they are used alone, like foods, sometimes for extended periods.

- **Herbal medicines can be used for modifying symptoms of disease and illness**, such as a deep cough where removal of mucous is necessary and can be addressed with expectorant herbs. High fevers can be lowered through the use of diaphoretic plants, which encourage sweating. Herbal medicines can help to ease symptoms, providing the body with some relief while enhancing immune system activity.
- **Plants offer a multitude of applications in the body for both internal and external support.** The skill of an herbalist is to know more than just one application for each plant, and you would do well to learn as much as you can about the multiple functions of the herbs you use. For example, yarrow is a bitter herb, therefore it has digestive tonic properties. Yet it is also a diaphoretic herb (increasing the body temperature and promoting sweating for a cold) and can be used as a menstrual tonic as well as a urinary antiseptic.
- **Herbs are often used in combination;** the synergistic action of the whole is more effective than using a single herb. In the case of herbs for high blood pressure, an effective formula frequently includes herbs for the management of fluid in the body, such as diuretics, as well as cardiovascular tonics, and relaxants to minimize stress and relax blood vessels, thereby lowering blood pressure. There are *main acting* herbs for organ systems and secondary *support herbs* that further aid the outcome of the blend by enhancing activity in related organ systems.
- **Individual chemicals versus whole herbs:** When herbs are taken in their whole form, they offer the most effective support for whole body health. Whole herb application utilizes hundreds of natural plant chemicals, many with synergistic properties that enhance the plant's overall efficacy and safety. By isolating one chemical obtained from a plant and altering it to a high concentration, one essentially creates an application closer in action to a pharmaceutical medication. For some plants, it is the synergistic activity, the multitude of constituents in the whole herb, that contributes to its many actions. For example, turmeric can be patented and marketed as a proprietary curcumin product, offering strong anti-inflammatory support. However, curcumin is just one of many curcuminoid compounds; by isolating and using just this one chemical from turmeric, one is missing out on the medicinal benefits obtained from numerous other chemicals contained within. These include volatile oils and nutrients (including beta

carotene, ascorbic acid (vitamin C), calcium, flavonoids, quercetin, azulene, turmerone, B vitamins and iron) and other curcuminoids (such as demethoxycurcumin, and bisdemethoxycurcumin).[28]

## Comparison Between a Pharmaceutical Drug and Herbal Medicine

The largest and perhaps most obvious difference between a plant and a pharmaceutical is that plants are alive just like us. They contain hundreds of complex chemical constituents, which work synergistically, and frequently offer buffering abilities from stronger active chemicals or contain chemicals that enhance the overall activity of an herb in our body. Plants are not as potent as prescriptions, so they take longer to work and they do not generally come with the same side effects.

Where pharmaceuticals are often used for just one effect in the body, herbal medicine involves a complex world of interdependent parts acting in more than one way. Many plants are known as "balancers" or "amphoteric" herbs, agents that bring the entire body back into equilibrium and assist in restoring homeostatic mechanisms.

# Safety and Dosage

Trained in plant medicine, I have come to trust the healing capacities of plants. Herbs are very safe when used respectfully. Some plants (and/or plant parts) are poisonous, and it is important to avoid these. Occasionally, though rare, individuals do have allergic reactions. However, to put this in perspective, some people react to relatively benign foods as well. The key is not to fear herbs; instead, recognize that they deserve our respect. When properly used, herbal medicines are highly efficient, and without the side effects of many prescription drugs and over the counter medications.

Sometimes, the application and efficacy of home remedies and self-treatment are limited by what we think we know to be true, or by incomplete information. If you are unsure about the causes of your disease or the proper remedies or applications, then seek a second or third opinion from a qualified health-care professional. When looking for information on herbal medicine, seek guidance from someone who is specifically trained in the field—a medical herbalist—or source out two to three excellent reference books written by herbalists in private practice.

Remember, you are the expert on your body. Listen to and trust the innate wisdom of your body. Use powerfully strong plants in smaller dosages. Try something and see how it feels. If a particular home treatment is not providing the desired results, then retrace your steps, double check your references, and obtain additional guidance from a health-care professional, ideally from one trained in holistic medicine. Remember that herbs work slower than fast-acting pharmaceuticals, and sometimes extremely gentle plants offer the most effective healing in the long run.

The herbs in this book are safe when taken within normal dosages. Some plants are more potent than others. If you are new to plant medicine, then some general guidelines will assist with your journey. Begin using a new plant at a lower dosage, and over a couple of days work up to the medicinal dose. If an adverse reaction should occur, then you will know.

Remember, however, that herbs can begin to remove congestion, promote cleansing, improve circulation, and shift digestive function; the first week may be more about the body adjusting to shifts in metabolism than actual adverse effects. If an application does not create the desired results, then there is a chance that symptoms have been misread. Consult a professional.

### Dosing

- A typical adult dosage for herbal tinctures, when taken internally, is one teaspoon taken three times per day. Let the herbs do their work at the suggested dosage. Unless an increase in dosage is recommended for acute conditions by a practicing herbalist, more is not necessarily better. More potent herbs are taken in smaller dosages. For acute conditions, like a cold or allergies, herbs can be taken more frequently. Because tinctures contain constituents from plants in a mixture of water and alcohol, it is recommended to dilute the tincture in hot water before drinking to evaporate much of the alcohol.
- Adult dosage for herbal teas: one teaspoon of herb per cup of hot water, taken three times per day, is a standard dosage.
- For the elderly, or individuals who are very sensitive or slim, a lower dose can often be used.
- The main area to be mindful of is pregnancy, to ensure safety for the baby (see Herbs to Avoid in Pregnancy on page 41). If you are pregnant, it is always advisable to obtain specific guidance from a health-care provider who can monitor your specific health issues, take into consideration the impact on the baby, and guide you accordingly. For infant dosage and application, refer to the guidelines in General Dosage Guidelines for Children on page 40.

Serious chronic illness should always be addressed through consultation with a health-care professional. If you are on numerous medications, it would be best to obtain guidance from one who can monitor you and ensure no contraindications rather than attempting to self-treat. Some pharmaceutical medications are very potent and can react with even the most normally mild foods. In any emergency situation, of course, head to a hospital for fast-acting, immediate treatment.

When discussing safety parameters, there is some need for common sense. If you have diarrhea or an irritable digestive tract, then don't reach for a strong herbal laxative unless you know what you are doing. Certain herbs may elevate blood pressure and therefore should be avoided in conditions of hypertension and/or glaucoma.

*"We are the ones we have been waiting for."* —Ghandi

## General Dosage Guidelines for Children

Almost all herbs suitable for adults can also be used for children. Remember, however, that children are smaller and so are their internal organs; adjust the dose accordingly for smaller weight and body size. Younger infants can also benefit from plant medicine; the very best administration route is through the mother's breast milk, thus having the mother consume three to five cups of tea depending on the situation. If this is not possible, the next best option is to prepare an herbal tea for a child's bathing water and use drop dosages with a dropper or syringe, following the age-dosage guidelines below.

**Young's Rule:**
Adult Dose x (Age ÷ (Age+12)) = Child's Dose

Example:
11 year old girl. Adult dose = 500mg.
500mg x (11 ÷ (11+12)) = Child's Dose
500mg x (11 ÷ 23) = Child's Dose
500mg x .48 = Child's Dose
Child's Dose = 240mg

**Cowling's Rule:**
Use the number of a child's next birthday and divide by 24.
For a child who is 5 years of age, soon to be 6, divide by 24 = 0.25 or one quarter the adult dose.

## Herbs to Avoid in Pregnancy

There are very few accounts of any herbs leading to adverse side effects during pregnancy, however it is responsible to consider a few general guidelines when pregnant. Avoid ingestion of any herbs that encourage menstruation (emmenagogues). Avoid ingestion of strong bitter herbs used to activate digestion, as they will also increase muscular contractions in the digestive tract, and avoid anti-parasitic and laxative herbs. These herbs are too stimulating to use. The very best advice is to consult an herbal practitioner for specific guidance when using any herbs during pregnancy. This is a list of some commonly-used western herbs that should not be ingested during pregnancy. Some herbs are dose- or circumstance-dependent and are not included in this list.

Arnica (*Arnica montana*)
Barberry (*Berberis vulgaris*)
Bayberry (*Myrica cerifera*)
Belladonna (*Atropa belladonna*)
Black cohosh (*Cimicifuga racemosa*)
Bloodroot (*Sanguinaria canadensis*)
Blue cohosh (*Caulophyllum thalictroides*)
Buchu (*Agathosma betulina*)
Chaparral (*Larrea divaricata*)
Coltsfoot (*Tussilago farfara*)
Comfrey (*Symphytum officinalis*)
Dong Quai (*Angelica sinensis*)
Feverfew (*Tanacetum parthenium*)
Ginseng (*Panax, Eleutherococcus*)
Goldenseal (*Hydrastis canadensis*)
Greater Celandine (*Chelidonium majus*)

Juniper (*Juniperus communis*)
Licorice (*Glycirrhiza glabra*)
Ma huang (*Ephedra sinica*)
Mistletoe (*Viscum album*)
Myrrh (*Commiphora molmol*)
Nutmeg (*Myristica fragrans*)
Parsley (*Petroselinum crispum*)
Pennyroyal (*Mentha pulegium*)
Poke Root (*Phytolacca decandra*)
Rue (*Ruta graveolens*)
Sage (*Salvia officinalis*)
Sassafras (*Sassafras albidum*)
Scotch broom (*Sarothamnus scoparius*)
Senna (*Cassia senna*)
Tansy (*Tanacetum vulgare*)
Tree of Life (*Thuja occidentalis*)
Wild Carrot (*Daucus carota*)
Wormwood (*Artemisia absinthium*)

# Preparation and Recommendations

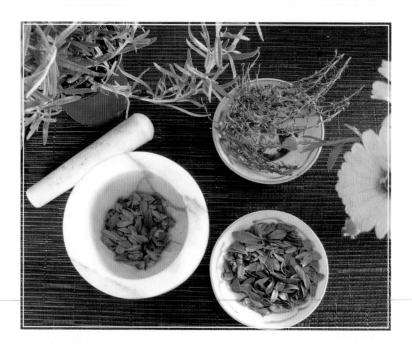

An herbalist's laboratory is the kitchen. Traditionally, the healing wisdom of plants was communicated by women while tending to the fire or during meal preparation. Recipes were passed on verbally or learned through observation of elders repeating applications for various ailments, from generation to generation. When teaching medicine-making classes, it is the sharing of personal stories, various outcomes, wisdom, and applications that brings the art of formulation to life. Everyone has a unique experience, and this is important to honor in the process.

Once the art of preparing herbal medicines has been mastered, there is vast room for creativity: exchanging ingredients, changing the flavor, choosing a more appropriate plant for a particular person (matching the personality of the plant with the needs of a particular person), selecting a local plant rather than ordering an exotic one, making a particular recipe more potent, increasing healing potential, and having fun with your creations. Some tips to keep in mind as you delve in: check your recipe more than once to confirm your inventory; pay attention to the emotions you bring into your medicine (this will be the maceration point of intentions: what you put in, you get back); infuse your medicine with the highest healing potential; and most importantly, the state where your mind rests will contribute to the quality of the medicine. Hold the highest outcome for effective medicine as your primary focus of intention, and thank the plants for their healing.

## Getting to Know Each Other

Take time to smell the roses. Get to know the visual appearance and aroma of each plant you are working with. This is an ideal way of beginning to meet the plant, so to speak, to get to know the unique flavors of their personality. Choose one plant at a time, and for a week or two observe its subtle actions. Write out the Latin names, and repeat them while using the medicine. Create your own cue cards when working with a specific plant until it is familiar; it's a lot like getting to know a person, gradually developing a relationship.

Taste the plants you are working with! Familiarize yourself with the unique flavors of various plants. Each one is unique. Let the flavors play on your palate—is the herb spicy, sweet, or pungent? One plant may summon the savoring of it in a cup of tea while the next selection may be bitter on your palate.

Observe how it feels in the body; knowing that this is your experience, honor it. Not everyone's experience will be similar. Feel how the body responds and build your confidence by connecting with your body's intuitive widsom.

## Obtaining Quality Herbs

Remember, the quality of the medicine is determined by the quality of ingredients selected. Grow your own organic plants or purchase high quality herbs from a local herb shop, choosing organic or sustainably wild-crafted plants when possible. The herbs should retain their original bright, vibrant color (hues should not be faded, leaves should be rich green, flowers should be their characteristic hue, and the plant should still hold its distinctive scent). Many plants contain volatile oils and can be identified just from their characteristic scent alone. For example, fennel, cinnamon, ginger, thyme, and spearmint can be recognized by their unique scent. Other plants just smell a friendly green. Dried herbs are at their most potent when used within a year of harvesting.

## Storage

Glass storage containers are an herbalist's best friend. Dark amber bottles can protect their contents from the damaging effects of sunlight. Otherwise, clear glass bottles with a secure-fitting lid, stored in a cupboard, will suffice. Store herbs in a cool, dry space—not the refrigerator, where moisture can be an issue. If you purchase an herb stored in plastic, transfer to a glass container and label it immediately. Many plants contain volatile oils or resins that start to leach out into the plastic, deteriorating the potency of the plant.

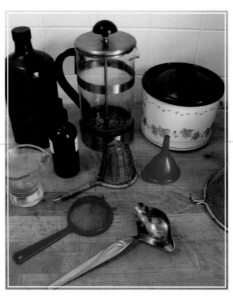

## Herbal Medicine–Making Equipment

Some of the most interesting medicine-making tools can be found very inexpensively at a local second hand shop or garage sale. Those wanting to make large volumes of medicine should look into obtaining a professional wine press (available in various sizes). Alternatively, a tea press or simple, hardy cotton can be used to manually (with the use of your muscles) separate out the plant material from liquid. Useful medicine-making tools include:

- Stainless steel funnels (Stainless steel is the best choice, as plastic ones can become sticky and difficult to clean.)
- Ladles for pouring into jars (I once found a steel ladle with spouts on either side which has been invaluable for medicine-making because it's ideal for both right-handed and left-handed individuals.)
- Containers like unique bottles, canning jars, and funky recycled glass are possible for home use (It is important to sterilize bottles to ensure a long shelf life and prevent contamination. Bottles can be sterilized by boiling for ten minutes or by running through the hot water cycle of a dishwasher. If a jar has a plastic insert, remove this as it can harbor bacteria.)
- Cheesecloth or cotton for straining
- Coffee grinder (Dedicated to herb grinding only—unless your goal is coffee-flavored medicine. Grind soft herbs only, or you'll risk burning out the motor of the grinder.)
- Strainers with various sizes of mesh
- Measuring cups
- Tea press or tea pot with strainer
- Cotton tea sacs of various sizes for brewing tea or baths
- Mortar and pestle
- Glass columns (graduated cylinders purchased from a science shop or pharmaceutical distribution company)
- Pruning shears, kitchen scissors, and sharp knife
- Double boiler
- Pots with lids (Ideal heating containers are stainless steel, ceramic, pyrex glass, cast iron, and enamel.)

- Slow cookers with three temperature settings (In my experience, slow cookers with only two temperature settings, low and high, can burn the medicine. Follow the Goldilocks principle: medium is just right!)

## Tips for Exceptional Medicine

*"You are the alchemist, who can invoke and channel the energy that pulsates above you, who can bring it down to earth and, in so doing, give it shape and form in accordance with your will and your intention." —Margot Anand*

Take time to prepare your creations—slow preparation time using low heat creates the best products. Do not burn your medicine. Heat is not your friend in this case, as it destroys heat-sensitive constituents.

Avoid the use of copper pots and aluminum for preparing medicines. Both metals can react with ingredients in the plant, altering the chemical properties and interfering with the potency of the medicine. Traces of aluminum may be found in the final product and the use of copper pots can destroy the vitamin C content in many herbs.

Ensure you have all ingredients and correct amounts prior to beginning. Pull out everything needed for a complete recipe and double check amounts. This will prevent you from being short a container or an ingredient for a recipe.

Create small batches for the first run, especially when making a new item or recipe for the first time.

Avoid the use of microwaves. Microwaves are also not your friend when preparing an herbal tea or any application. Use a kettle to boil water, and take the time to reheat tea on the stove rather than destroying the plant constituents.

Reference two or three very precise medicine-making texts, and get to know the function and action of each ingredient in a recipe. If just beginning to create your potions and elixirs at home, you will be grateful to compare the various preparation options and descriptions. Read the handbooks over in detail and compare and contrast information for a solid foundation of application.

## Labeling

Sound like an overrated section? I cannot say enough about the importance of detailed labeling. Label all items as soon as possible or risk omitting valuable information for duplicating the medicine in the future. For herbal recipes, record the name and intention of the medicine, preparation date, directions, ingredients, and strength (proportions of herbs or ratio of liquid to herbs and percentage of alcohol). Have fun creating your own stunning homemade labels by using a calligrapher's pen and colored ink by hand or choose a fun font on the computer.

For single herbs: record both the Latin and common name, date harvested, and (if you have this information) the date received and best before date. List actions, directions, and any cautions.

### Where to Begin

Begin your journey with plant medicine one herb at a time. Begin the relationship just like meeting a new friend for the first time. Relationships take time for familiarity to build, as it takes time to notice subtleties in the personality of each plant. Like the colorful personalities of each person, plants also have their own unique quirks and preferences.

Reference two to three herbal medicine books (preferably written by herbalists, not someone from another paradigm) and create your own personal file cards on each herb, listing various actions, applications, preparations and harvesting tips. Take time to sit with the plant, observing its choice of home and characteristics in nature. Observe it growing, draw it, spend time with it. Get to know its growing preferences, harvest it if possible, prepare it in a tea and allow its taste to dance on the tongue. Sample a tincture and observe any immediate body responses. Is the herb bitter in taste? Notice the release of saliva in the mouth? Notice how the herb activates the digestive juices throughout the digestive tract, beginning with the letdown response of saliva and release of digestive enzymes, amylase, and lipase in the mouth. It is valuable to note that bitter plant properties are also ideal for topical applications, for example as skin washes for stubborn infections and open wounds.

# HERBS IN THE KITCHEN

Just as a chef can list ten or more ways to sauté an onion, an herbalist knows numerous healing properties of plants for various ills. Most people can identify one use for Echinacea—its application for colds. Can you list five more applications or traditional uses? Therein lies the skill of an herbalist.

Open up the spice drawer. Many common kitchen spices, and even vegetables found in the crisper, contain medicinal properties. Caraway, cinnamon, cumin, black pepper, ginger, turmeric, onion, cabbage, potato, carrot, rosemary, oregano, sage, basil, and thyme are all effective therapeutic medicines. Horseradish, perhaps better known in the culinary world as an ingredient often found in wasabi, is certainly a spicy condiment, but it is also one of nature's potent medicines. The difference between medicine versus simple food comes down to understanding the full potential of healing properties of the plant, knowing the correct application routes and dosages, and having the skill to apply this information for the desired results. Have fun with your creations!

## Mustard Seeds

Also known as white or black mustard, the white being the milder of the two, mustard seed varieties include brown, Indian mustard, and others. Mustard seed or seed powder is used medicinally as a valuable member of the cabbage or *Brassicaceae* family.

**Constituents:** glycosides (mustard oils), glucosinolates (sinigrin, precursor to allyl isothiocyanate, which has anti-microbial and anti-fungal properties), glucoraphanin (the chemical precursor to sulforaphane, an anti-cancer property and the focus of much research), flavonoids, fixed oils, proteins (amino acids), mucilage, bitter principles and enzymes are just a few chemical constituents present.[29]

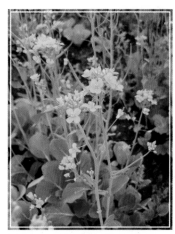

**Mustard Seeds (*Brassica nigra* and *alba*) Family: *Brassicaceae***

**Medicinal Actions:** diaphoretic, circulative tonic, rubefacient, antifungal

**Applications:** plaster, poultice or liniment, footbath, body soak, and a welcome condiment

Yes, this is the same mustard used as a condiment in sandwiches. Reach for this valued medicine for symptoms associated with respiratory congestion and for relief during the cold and flu season.

Today mustard is mainly used as a topical application. It works as a diaphoretic, meaning it increases the blood flow to the peripheries, or locally on the skin, and stimulates sweating, thereby reducing a high body temperature.

Prepare these traditional mustard packs for bronchial congestion, phlegmy coughs and pneumonia. They ease the pain of arthritic joints, sore muscles, and sciatica. Mix the mustard powder with water to form a thick paste. Another option includes substituting apple cider vinegar for water. Place into cotton or muslin and apply a thin layer of cream or oil barrier between the skin and the mustard pack, especially for a child. Apply the pack to the skin (chest for a cold, a joint for arthritic support). Remember though, this is an herb to respect! It is heating! If too hot and left for too long, it can cause the skin to blister!

The term "rubefacient," also known as a counterirritant, refers to when a heating agent like mustard is applied to the skin and stimulates fresh blood flow to a localized area, inviting heat to local tissues. As blood vessels dilate and circulation is increased, more blood is drawn to local tissues, sending enhanced healing properties and nutrients into the blood. The anti-inflammatory nature of rubefacients is thought to work through a reflex action mediated by the nervous system.

Mustard is warming to our extremities as well as our insides. It supports digestion and is used to negate gas and bloating. How many of us remember mustard as a condiment from childhood days (hot dogs on a bun—or in today's era, veggie dogs)? The herb is best used in powder form, as a paste. Alternatively, if you appreciate mustard, pick the fresh herb greens with their delicious yellow flowers to add some depth to salads, stews, salad dressings or meat marinades.

Prepare a footbath containing mustard powder, or add in crushed seeds to warm up cold hands and feet after frolicking outdoors in blizzard winter weather! This would be an ideal first aid application for hypothermia, however it is certainly effective to use for instantly heating up those cold hands and feet.

### Warming Mustard Foot Bath

Two tablespoons of mustard powder and one tablespoon grated ginger root into a warm footbath, adding five drops of eucalyptus essential oil to ease cold or sore, aching muscles associated with a flu (or instead prepare a sinus steam to encourage draining of congestion from the sinuses).

### Tips for Topical Use

- Protect the skin with a thin layer of cream or oil or muslin.
- Use for a short time and test the temperature.
- If pronounced redness occurs, rub in a carrier oil such as grape-seed, almond or even olive oil to provide relief.
- For internal use, condiment dosages are certainly safe for this warming herb. Keep in mind that this is a stronger herb, so avoid ingestion of high amounts. Its acrid taste alone could lead to vomiting.

## Horseradish Root

Another valued medicine from the same Cabbage family, horseradish is known as Mountain Radish. The root, used as the medicinal part, is harvested in autumn and prepared fresh.

**Constituents:** volatile oils—glucosinolates: mustard oil glycosides, (sinigrin, as it mixes with water, yields mustard oil[30]), asparagine, resin, vitamin C, B vitamins.[31] Mustard oil is a sulphur-containing compound that is warming and possesses antimicrobial and antibacterial properties.

All of the nutrient values to follow have been referenced from the USDA National Nutrient Database:

Mustard Greens: 100 g delivers 115 mg Calcium, 1.64 mg Iron, 32 mg Magnesium, and 70 mg Vitamin C[32]

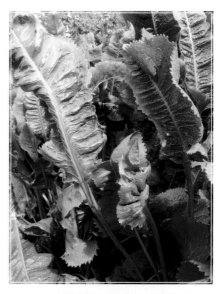

**Horseradish Root (*Cochlearia armoracia* and *Armoracia rusticana*) Family: *Brassicaceae***

Mustard Seed, ground: 1 tablespoon delivers 17 mg Calcium, and 23 mg Magnesium[33]

It is another example of a condiment with medicinal properties. Use just a little to be effective! Have you tasted sushi? Recall the effects of horseradish containing wasabi directly on the tongue. For me, the effect is an instant head rush with sinus clearing, saliva increasing, and nose running effects. A dramatic reaction! This herb packs a whole lot of potency in a small serving. Only a small amount is needed.

**Medicinal Actions:** antiseptic, anticatarrhal, warming circulatory stimulant, digestive, carminative

**Applications:** condiment, liniment, herbal vinegar, syrup, skin wash, poultice

Reach for wasabi or use fresh grated horseradish root mixed with a small amount of water in external preparations for its anticatarrhal (mucus-moving) properties, to remove congestion and excess phlegm from the lungs. The root contains glucosinolates and mustard oils (creating a pungent taste), which enhance its warming and antimicrobial properties.

Mustard oils are quickly absorbed into the skin and digestive tract and are eliminated from the body via the respiratory tract and kidneys. As the oils exit, they become antiseptic. The glucosinolates, particularly asparagine, are excreted through the kidneys, contributing to the diuretic effect and assisting removal of uric acid from the urine.

When applied topically as a tea or liniment, these antiseptic benefits can be used for washing an infection, promoting tissue healing, or bleeding wounds.

Like ginger, cinnamon, cayenne, and other heating spices, when ingesting horseradish, the effects are quick to see through improved peripheral circulation and the rise in healing qualities as part of the improved blood flow. As blood flow increases, a rise in body temperature, sweating, and a sense of warmth also occurs. When outdoors in cold temperatures, it provides warming support for winter chills, colds, and hands that never warm up completely (even hypothermia).

A horseradish root puree can be packed into a poultice. Add lukewarm (rather than hot) water to moisten, place a carrier oil between you and this warming herb, and apply to the chest for bronchitis and congestion. Reach for horseradish for tissue regeneration, for slow healing wounds and to increase the flow of blood to local tissues, sending more nutrients and healing properties to the area.

This is another rubefacient heating herb that creates local flushing and redness like a mustard pack, increasing the rate of healing and sending more nutrients to the tissues. Apply to ease stiffness and muscle aches and to heal tissue. Reach for this topical analgesic when you would consider applying heat for relief.

**Take note:** Horseradish may have the potential to slow down thyroid function, so consider using horseradish as a condiment if you are experiencing an overactive thyroid. Do not ingest large amounts during pregnancy and lactation.

**Mindfulness:** Horseradish is one of those herbs that nature created on the spicy side to limit its palatability and ingestion. Overconsumption is highly unlikely due to the potent, biting nature of this hot-tasting herb, and it requires only logic to ingest what dose is bearable as a condiment. Let your taste buds be your guide!

Horseradish is spicy, so be sure to avoid when there is stomach inflammation or ulceration.

It should be used as an occasional food or medicine, not consumed in copious amounts. Over-ingestion may lead to vomiting and diarrhea. The adult dosage should not exceed more than two to three grams of fresh root two to three times daily.[34]

If you ever decide to eat it right off the spoon, then know that horseradish becomes more palatable when taken with honey. Tea or tincture can also be effective in very small dosages, though not very palatable.

Horseradish is an amazing herb containing antiseptic properties, with a special affinity for the respiratory tract and circulation enhancement. Reach for the Plague blend, below, in the winter months. One taste of this mixture and the effects are apparent: a clearing of sinuses during congestion, an antiseptic circulatory stimulant for cold hands and feet, allergies, and to help alleviate the chills of a cold.

# HOT AND SPICY HORSERADISH PLAGUE BLEND

## Ingredients
1 cup peeled and cubed fresh Horseradish root
1 Shallot
1 Garlic clove, crushed
2 cups Apple Cider Vinegar
½ teaspoon Turmeric root powder
½ teaspoon Ginger root powder
¼ teaspoon Cayenne Pepper powder
½ teaspoon Thyme herb
½ teaspoon Oregano herb
½ teaspoon Cinnamon Bark (or powder)
A grind or two of Peppercorns
Honey

## Directions
Add horseradish in a blender or food processor with the shallot and garlic. Blend. Add apple cider vinegar and spices. Blend until slightly choppy. If the desired effect is a smooth pureed mixture, then add in a teaspoon of water until desired consistency is reached. Add in honey to taste. Store in fridge and use as a condiment, or take directly on the spoon for immune support and chronic sinus infections—use up within 4 weeks. This is not the most palatable medicine, yet it is very effective.

## Cabbage

In Latin, the Brassicaceae or *Brassica* family, directly translates to "cabbage" or cabbage family, referring to the whole valuable group of nutrient-rich cruciferous vegetables, including cabbage, broccoli, kale, kohlrabi, collard greens, cauliflower, bok choy, mustard greens, watercress, and brussel sprouts.

There are numerous varieties of cabbage, including red, green, savoy, bok choy, and napa (Chinese) cabbage, all of which can be used interchangeably. However, red cabbage has higher anti-inflammatory properties and a higher nutritional profile, while bok choy is reputed to have the mildest flavor. This round or oval leafy vegetable has soft leaves that can be peeled off of the

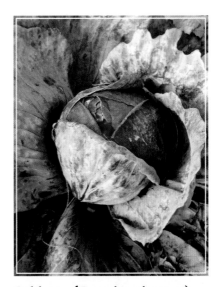

**Cabbage (*Brassica oleracea*) Family: *Brassicaceae***

inner core and used as medicine. To an herbalist, the numerous health benefits are impressive. Cabbage, in my estimation, is clearly a superfood.

Cabbage contains some of the highest amounts of antioxidants found in cruciferous vegetables: (including thiocyanates, lutein, zeaxanthin, isothiocyanates), polyphenols, glucosinolates (sulforaphane and indole-3-carbinol, which both stimulate liver detoxification), and carotenoids.[35] Anthocyanins are found in purple cabbage.

Cabbage has both antibiotic and anti-irritant properties. It contains sinigrin (allyl isothiocyanate), rapine, mustard oil, magnesium, oxylate, and sulphur heterosides. Its constituents help to decrease tissue congestion by dilating local small blood vessels, improving the blood flow in the area.

**Medicinal actions:** obesity, cleansing detoxifier, liver health, antiseptic, gout, mastitis, bowel health, high-fiber food, anti-inflammatory for rheumatism and arthritis, antioxidant

**Applications:** nutritive food, poultice, fomentation, vinegar

Cabbage supports digestion, stomach health, and is an ideal source of fiber, containing 3.3 grams per 100 grams. It increases bulk in the stools for regularity of bowel function, reducing constipation, and works to create a more alkaline body. Add cabbage into a diet where cleansing and detoxification is needed to assist the removal of waste from the stomach and bowels as well as uric acid from the kidneys. Also, cabbage can be included in the diet for conditions of gout, arthritis, kidney stones, and skin eruptions.

Traditional recipes consider cabbage an amazing remedy for the entire digestive system, improving nutrient assimilation and gut healing. It is considered one of the best foods for ulcers. Ingest fresh green cabbage juice daily for stomach and duodenal ulcers and for excess acidity in the digestive system. A traditional remedy used by the late Dr. Vogel in his book *The Nature Doctor* combined raw potato juice before meals with cabbage juice after meals for healing ulcers.[36] Today we understand that cabbage contains L glutamine, an amino acid, a gut healer, and an essential nutrient for maintenance of healthy intestinal cells, preventing leaky gut or increased intestinal permeability. The antioxidants and glucosinolates can help to ensure healthy gut bacteria, even lowering the risk of H. pylori (*Helicobacter pylori* in the stomach).

If straight cabbage juice is simply not agreeable to your palate, then add the juice into a soup or stew to mask the taste and find ways to add both raw and steamed cabbage into your diet.

Cabbage (and all cruciferous vegetables actually) has been the subject of much research in the area of cancer prevention. A quick search on Google scholar shows 42,200 results on the topic of cabbage and cancer; similarly, on PubMed, over 700 abstracts were available at the time of writing this book. Studies indicate the cancer preventive properties of cabbage are threefold:

1. Offering benefit through its long known anti-inflammatory properties
2. Providing high antioxidant levels[37]
3. Containing high amounts of chemicals called glucosinolates, which may support liver detoxification

Antioxidant compounds in cabbage may offer protection against several types of cancer, including breast, colon, bladder, and prostate cancers.[38,39,40,41] The glucosinolates help improve the body's ability to detoxify and eliminate harmful chemicals, pollutants and assist in eliminating excess circulating hormones, indicating value in fighting hormone-dependent cancers.[42] Studies are indicating that glucosinolates in cabbage, including sulforaphane and indole-3-carbinole (I3C) can help increase the rate of estrogen breakdown occurring in the liver,[43,44,45] supporting the fact that cabbage can offer some protective properties against estrogen-dependent breast cancer and other hormone-driven cancers.

I have obtained some of the greatest insights on healing from reading herbal texts of the early twentieth century. Dr. Alfred Vogel also combines raw potato and cabbage as a poultice for healing wounds[46] and mixes in carrot juice as a daily tonic recipe for easing symptoms of gout and arthritis. Cabbage has a history of topical application for swelling and joint pain related to arthritis, both consuming it internally and using the grated leaves in a topical poultice to wrap around the joints. The polyphenols found in all cabbage provide marked anti-inflammatory support for the body; however, reach for red cabbage for strongest antioxidant and anti-inflammatory compounds.[47]

For mastitis and breast engorgement, occasionally encountered by breast-feeding mothers, cabbage leaves come to the rescue. An effective approach for reducing the pain and swelling is to take a cabbage leaf, crush or bruise the leaf slightly (roll the leaf under a rolling pin to release more of the healing properties), and place it into the cup of a bra. Ensure the leaf covers the breast. After a couple hours the leaf will be wilted. Replace with a fresh leaf and repeat throughout the day. At night, replace the wilted leaf with a fresh one and sleep with the leaf on overnight. Repeat until engorgement subsides.

**Note:** This application works very well for breast engorgement but may decrease milk production during its application. If this occurs, then support the body through using the lactation promotion tea on page 66.

- **For skin afflictions such as eczema, psoriasis, acne, rashes, insect bites, bruising, and leg ulcers:** prepare a poultice.
- **For stubborn boils:** prepare a poultice or wash to bring the boil to a head.
- **As a wound healer and for arthritic joints:** prepare a topical application.
- **For bleeding gums and gingivitis:** prepare fresh cabbage juice.
- **For pimples, drying acne, or other skin irritations:** the juice or poultice of cabbage can be applied to the skin.
- **For healthier hair and nails:** use the fresh juice as a rinse for hair, and a nutritive food ingested internally for nails.
- Take note! Cabbage juice is one of the best hangover remedies!

# Traditional Hair Growth Application

**Ingredients**
1 cup Cabbage, chopped and boiled (or 1 cup Cabbage juice)
Juice of ½ Lemon
2–3 drops Rosemary Essential Oil

**Directions**
Boil or juice cabbage, remove from heat, and add the juice of one freshly-squeezed lemon and rosemary essential oil. Place in a blender to form a thick paste. Massage into scalp and roots and let stand for 30 minutes. Shampoo and condition hair. Repeat 2–3 times per week to stimulate scalp circulation and promote growth of silky shiny hair.

# Indo Cabbage Sauté

## Ingredients
2 tablespoons Coconut Oil
1 Onion, finely chopped
1 teaspoon Mustard seeds
1 teaspoon Mustard powder
1 tablespoon Turmeric powder
Liberal shakes of Cayenne powder
1 teaspoon fresh grated Ginger
½ cup Water
4 cups Red Cabbage, shredded
1 teaspoon Salt
Raisins, presoaked in water (although at the time of sampling my creation, no raisins were found, so I used dried Juniper berries instead. Delicious!)
Gomashio or Sunflower seeds
Sesame oil can be drizzled over top for a savory eastern flavor

## Directions
Heat oil in a skillet over medium heat, add onion and spices; sauté for 1 minute. Stir in water and shredded cabbage; add salt and raisins. Cover and steam until cabbage is soft but not mushy. Remove from heat, then sprinkle sunflower seeds or gomashio (sesame seasoning) over top. Serve either hot or cold. Consuming warm offers amazing immediate relief for bronchial congestion while improving circulation to the body.

## Safety Profile
Ingesting large quantities of uncooked raw cabbage *may* slow down the thyroid's uptake of iodine, and therefore may interfere with the thyroid gland's ability to convert T4 to the more active T3.[48] Thus, if you are experiencing an underactive thyroid condition, the ingestion of raw cruciferous vegetables should be limited. Cooking seems to deactivate this effect.

## Watercress

The pungent, peppery flavor reminds us that this plant is also found in the mustard family. The Latin name is derived from the words *nasus tortus*, meaning a convulsed nose, of course referring to the slightly pungent, spicy mustard scent and flavor of the leafy greens.

The whole herb is used medicinally. Be certain to wash this tender herb well before ingestion. I personally use a vegetable wash to soak the plant and to ensure that the *only* thing being ingested is the watercress.

**Constituents:** flavonoids (quercetin), sulfur compounds, glucosinolates, isothiocyanates, carotenoids, lutein, iodine[49]

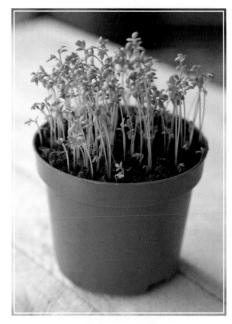

**Watercress (*Nasturtium officinale*) Family: *Brassicaceae***

Watercress is a valuable tonic to build the blood. Consider combining with carrots and spinach for enhanced mineral content. For every 100 g of plant material, there are 43 mg of Vitamin C, 120 g of Calcium, 330 ml Potassium, and 3,191 IU of Vitamin A.[50]

**Medicinal Actions**: antiseptic expectorant, cholagogue, antioxidant and nutritive, lung tonic

**Applications:** nutritious food, fresh juice, broth, infusion

Known as a detoxifying and body-purifying spring tonic, watercress is packed full of vitamins and minerals. It has been said to cleanse the blood and strengthen the body. Typically, it is used in the spring to remove toxins accumulated during the winter months and for mild constipation. An alkaline tonic for acidic conditions such as arthritis, gout, and rheumatism, it is also used to improve the appetite, warm the stomach, nourish the entire body, and to stimulate liver and gallbladder function. Use as a food, tea, or tincture.

Being a member of the cabbage family, watercress also contains glucosinolates and high amounts of antioxidant nutrients, making this food a useful immune and possible anticancer nutrient. From laboratory and in vitro studies, animal models to some human research, studies indicate that isothiocyanates in cruciferous vegetables can inhibit cancer development by activating the ability of phase II liver enzymes (such as glutathione S transferases) to detoxify.[51] They can also stimulate apoptosis (selective cancer cell death), and may inactivate nitrosamine carcinogens in mice studies by inhibiting specific cytochrome P450 enzymes.[52,53] Finally, they may assist in the regulation of normally uncontrolled growth of cancer cells.[54,55]

As a lung tonic, watercress can be used as a food staple to strengthen the lungs, removing congestion and excess phlegm, for bronchitis or regular smoking.

- **For spider bites:** prepare a poultice from steamed watercress.
- **A relief for hemorrhoids:** prepare a poultice from steamed watercress.
- **For skin spots and freckles:** the fresh watercress juice can be applied directly on spots, wrinkles, and freckles.
- **A topical application for eczema:** apply as juice or poultice.

**Tea:** infusion with fresh or dried watercress and ingested as needed.

The juice of fresh watercress can be taken internally, added into a smoothie or soup, or used externally on the skin. One to two ounces of fresh juice is all that is needed as a daily tonic.

**Nutrition:** Soak the watercress in water before use. Watercress can be chopped and added into a salad, soups, or minced and sprinkled on vegetables. A delicious addition to potatoes, add in the minced watercress greens before mashing. Use instead of lettuce: layer it into a traditional sandwich or steam and sauté, serving like you would spinach. Add to omelettes or frittatas.

**Caution:** Although very rare and certainly not typically noted in culinary cookbooks, when watercress leaves are not cleaned properly, there is a small risk of contamination with the ova from a liver fluke, Fascioliasis, causing liver issues in humans.[56] So purchasing watercress from a market (where the watercress has been grown in fresh water and sand), rather than risking a wild harvest from a possibly contaminated water source, is always the best option and ensures the highest safety.

# Spring Cleansing Mineral-Rich Watercress Broth

## Ingredients

2 tablespoons Extra Virgin Olive Oil or Coconut Oil
1 medium Onion, coarsely chopped into cubes
6 cups Water
2 medium Carrots, diced
2 stalks Celery, diced
1 fresh root Gobo (Burdock), peeled and diced (when in season),
or 2 tablespoons dried root
1 medium Zucchini, diced
2 cloves Garlic, minced
Kelp powder, season to taste
1 teaspoon Turmeric powder
Black Pepper powder to season
4 cups Watercress (1 bunch), washed well and chopped
2 cups young Nettle leaves (when in season); wash well while wearing
    gloves, chop finely
1 bunch Parsley, finely chopped
2 tablespoons finely chopped Cilantro
1 medium Beet, grated
*Optional: add in medicinal mushrooms like shiitake, maitake, or oyster for
    additional immune support.

## Directions

Sauté the onion in oil in a pot on the stove until yellow. Add in water and
bring to a boil. Reduce heat to a simmer. Add in carrots, celery, gobo, zucchini, garlic, and seasoning. Slowly simmer until vegetables are tender but
not mushy. Add in chopped watercress, nettles, parsley, cilantro, and grated
beets and let sit for 5 minutes, covered, before serving.

# Pink Grapefruit, Watercress, and Goat Feta Salad

## Ingredients

1 Red Onion, finely sliced
1 bunch Watercress, tough stem ends removed and well washed
    (about 4 cups)
1 Avocado, cubed
¼ cup Pumpkin seeds, unsalted
1 Ruby Red Grapefruit
Coarse ground Black Pepper
4 tablespoons fresh Tarragon herb
1 tablespoon Apple Cider Vinegar
1 tablespoon Olive Oil
Cayenne pepper powder
1/3 cup Goat Feta, crumbled
Substitution: Ripe watermelon or orange slices can also be used instead of
    grapefruit, and try substituting fresh mint leaves for a variation in flavor.

## Directions

Combine onion, watercress, avocado, and pumpkin seeds in a bowl. Slice off
the top and bottom of the grapefruit and peel each segment using a sharp
knife. Cut off the skin, removing any white pith (which is nutritious but will
contribute to a bitter taste in the salad). Squeeze the skin and grapefruit
membranes to release any remaining juice and add this into the salad mixture. Toss in black pepper, tarragon, vinegar, olive oil, and cayenne pepper;
crumble in feta cheese and serve.

## Fennel Seed

An aromatic herb with yellow flowers and hard rigid seeds, fennel is known by many local names such as wild fennel, common, sweet fennel, bitter, roman and fennel of Florence. Its seeds and leaves are used medicinally. Use the root bulb as a delicious ingredient for cooking. Its sweet, warm, aromatic scent is fabulous sautéed or steamed with other herbs and vegetables.

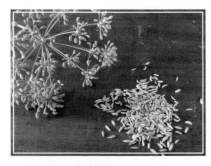

**Fennel Seed (*Foeniculum officinalis*) Family: *Apiaceae***

**Chemical Constituents:** volatile oil (anethole, limonene and others), phenolic acids, flavonoids, coumarins, sterols, fixed oils.[57] One tablespoon of Fennel seed provides 69 mg of Calcium, 1.08 mg of Iron, and 22 mg of Magnesium, 98 mg of Potassium, and 8 IU of Vitamin A.[58]

**Medicinal Actions:** carminative, galactagogue, expectorant for chronic coughs, anti-colic, stomachic, anti-inflammatory

**Applications:** infusion, tincture, cooking, syrup, gripe water, vinegar, essential oil

The lactation tonic (also known by the term "galactagogue" to herbalists), Fennel has had centuries of safe, traditional use for its ability to increase the secretion of breast milk in new mothers. This is dose-dependent. If the milk is not flowing after delivery, then begin drinking four to five cups of fennel tea, and give it a couple of days for the effects of fennel to begin working. My clients' feedback tells me this tea works like a charm and is without the concerning side effects of the pharmaceutical lactation stimulant medications (instead, fennel tea may also help reduce the likelihood of colic in your infant and gently calm an upset tummy).

Have you heard of gripe water? An over the counter pharmaceutical option for infant's colic, you will find various recipes with active ingredients listed as fennel, ginger, or dill. Then look at the full ingredient list, including the non-medicinal ingredients, depending upon the brand. In addition to the actives, the formula may contain syrup (consisting of sucrose or fructose), sodium and potassium benzoate (which may form benzene, a known carcinogen), polysorbate 80 (linked with many health risks including breathing difficulties, blood clots, irregular heartbeat, fainting, fever, allergic reactions,[59] and possibly predispose to Crohn's and colitis,[60,61]) sime-thicone (some generic brands contain aluminum), parabens, and alcohol. Why feed a newborn all of these unnecessary additives? Consider simply choosing the main ingredient and preparing as a tea for outstanding results.

Prepared as an infusion, this subtle licorice-scented herb is known as a carminative, a soothing digestive for gas, bloating. Its anti-inflammatory and anti-spasmodic properties gently calm a spastic bowel and soothe colic and digestive upsets in infants as well as calm spasms due to coughs. Add in small amounts to any respiratory or digestive tea blend as a flavor enhancer with medicinal properties. Consider this a go-to herb for digestive distress. Fennel is known as an expectorant herb, one that loosens and assists the removal of phlegm from the lungs. Prepare a tea and bathe a young infant or use a syringe and use drop dosages as provided on page 40.

The bulb can be thinly sliced and used as an appetizer, sautéed with onion, or steamed as part of a mixed vegetable dish or chutney.

**Cautions:** For people allergic to the carrot or celery families, occasionally dermatitis and respiratory allergies may occur, though I have never seen this in clinical practice.

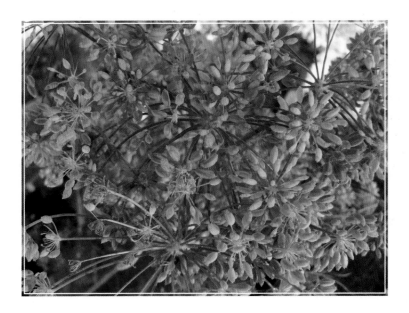

# Fennel Mother's Milk Tea

## Ingredients
2 parts Fennel seed
2 parts Caraway seed
1 part Nettle leaf
1 part Chickweed herb

## Directions
This is a gentle-tasting tea with mild fennel flavors and the subtle aroma of caraway. Mix herbs together and store in a glass container with a tight-fitting lid. Use 2 heaping tablespoons of tea mixture to 2 cups of water. Pour boiling water over the herbs. Cover and steep for 15 minutes. Strain and drink 4–5 cups per day to encourage the letdown of milk.

## Carrot Root

**Common names of Carrot include:** Bee's nest plant, Bird's nest, Queen Anne's lace and Wild carrot.

Carrot is a plant growing two to four feet tall. It is used as a food—with the bright orange root in the cultivated carrots we know as root vegetables—and the seeds from the wild carrot are used medicinally. The seeds are harvested in early autumn for the wild variety, and the cultivated variety with the edible orange root is harvested in late fall. Carrot leaf has been used as an edible green, consumed in low amounts.

Wild carrot is commonly known by herbalists as Queen Anne's lace or bird's nest plant. It is found along roadsides, grassy areas, cliffs, and coastal areas.

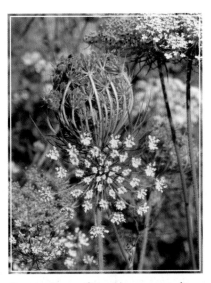

**Carrot Root (*Daucus carota*)
Family: *Apiaceae***

It is distinguishable by the unique bird's nest-like lacy white flower clusters, each with five petals. It has one small purple, red or black floret at the center. It blooms from April to October. The seeds are of a dull brown color yet fragrantly scented, flat on one side and convex on the other. If the root is pulled up, it will have the characteristic aroma of carrots, and you will discover a yellow-white, tough, woody root, thinner than cultivated garden carrots yet edible.

**Chemical Constituents (from fruit or seeds):** flavonoids (apigenin, luteolin, quercetin), volatile oil, daucine, fatty acids, coumarin, xylitol[62] and other constituents, polyphenols, polyacetylenes (falcarinol, falcarindiol—contributing to the bitter taste), myristicin, and carotenoids (beta-carotene and lutein).

The bright orange-red roots of Carrots are packed full of nutrients, 100 g offers 16 706 IU of Vitamin A, 19 ug of Folate, 33 mg Calcium, 12 mg Magnesium, 320 mg Potassium, and 2.8 grams of dietary Fiber.[63]

**Medicinal Actions:** diuretic, deobstruent, anthelmintic, carminative, stimulant, galactagogue, ophthalmic (referring to eye health), digestive tonic, diuretic, emmenagogue

**Applications:** nutritive food, fresh juice, infusion, poultice, hair rinse, body care

According to Mrs. Grieve, in her book *The Modern Herbal*, carrot seeds were traditionally used for their carminative properties of benefit for digestive issues, dysentery, colic, and coughs.[64]

**Eye health:** Carrots contain beta-carotene and lutein, which is converted in the body to vitamin A, useful for night vision and protection against macular degeneration and development of cataracts.[65]

Adding carrots (as well as those cruciferous vegetables) into your diet may play a role in cancer prevention.[66] Research shows that the naturally-occurring antioxidants (including beta-carotene and lutein) and another chemical called Falcarinol, a natural anti-fungal chemical found in carrots, may offer cancer protection properties.[67,68,69]

This antioxidant rich food offers protection for the lungs and protection from infections. Individuals experiencing breathing difficulties such as emphysema, bronchitis, and smoker's lungs should consider incorporating carrots into their diet.

Carrot roots are an alkaline-cleansing food and nourisher known to encourage the body's detox capacities and reduce acidic conditions. It is considered a deobstrucient, which means it removes barriers and obstacles from the body's normal functioning. Carrots help normalize digestive function; their fiber is useful for colon health, working to regulate digestive imbalances, conditions such as diarrhea and constipation, heartburn, and excess stomach acidity. Research shows that carrot extracts can offer gentle liver protective properties.[70] Consider steamed carrots as gentle tonics for those who are weak after illness and those who are dealing with congestion and toxic load. It even offers internal cleansing for skin blemishes and acne.

- **Gas, colic and stomach inflammation:** prepare carrot seed tea infusion.
- **Parasite prevention and remedy:** grate raw carrots as a home remedy (used along with raw pumpkin seeds) to help expel worms in children.
- **Anemia:** consume fresh carrot juice to assist with building the blood.
- **Dandruff:** prepare a hair rinse for a dry, flaking scalp using fresh carrot juice.
- **Damaged Skin:** carrots and carrot oil can be used in body care recipes for dry, aging, sun-damaged skin and broken capillaries.
- **For burns:** prepare a poultice of raw carrots to soothe the skin.

Carrot juice offers anti-allergy support and can assist with decreasing excess phlegm and congestion from the upper respiratory tract, easing nasal congestion.

Perhaps the most traditional application for carrots relates to their diuretic action and for stimulating the removal of waste material from the kidneys. Traditionally, they have been used for chronic urinary tract issues, cystitis, gout, and fluid retention. Carrot seeds are considered anti-lithic (an agent helping to prevent or clear stones and gravel from the kidneys and for symptoms of painful voiding). Carrot leaves can be used for gout (add into salads and daily juicing recipes).

Wild carrot seeds have been used for centuries as a contraceptive.[71] However, any reliance on this information is done solely at your own discretion; research this in more depth prior to trying (I suggest seeking out an herbalist in your area who is familiar with the application of use). Infusion of carrot seeds can provide assistance for menstrual cramps and promote the onset of menstruation.

Ensure proper plant identification! It's crucial if harvesting wild carrots, as there are other very similar-looking plants that are poisonous. Do not mistake wild carrot for poison hemlock (a hairless replica). Only harvest wild carrots if you are absolutely certain of the correct identification of species, as misidentification can be fatal. If ever in doubt, do not harvest. Instead, seek out someone who can offer a confirmation of species, and always double check your facts.

## Comparison Chart: Wild Carrot and Poison Hemlock

References from *Edible Wild Food* online at www.ediblewildfood.com and HubPages article by Leah Lefler, "How to Identify Queen Anne's Lace (Wild carrot)."

### Wild Carrot
- Keep your eyes open for a purple "heart" in the center of the flowers (which could be pink, dark red, or black).
- Carrots are smaller, growing two to three feet.
- Queen Anne's lace goes to seed, with the umbels folding up, almost resembling a bird's nest (one of its common names).
- The seeds of the Queen Anne's lace have spiny structures on the outside and fine hairs on the solid green stems.
- When the leaves are crushed, they have the scent of carrots.

### Poisonous Hemlock
- The scent is a musky, putrid smell like parsnips.
- The stems are hairless.
- There is no small, dark flower in the center.
- It is a larger plant, growing up to eight feet in height.
- Poison hemlock flower clusters do not fold up.
- Poison hemlock seeds are smooth.
- When hemlock goes to seed, it produces small brown seeds on its umbels.
- Hemlock has smooth stems, and the lower portion of the stem will be streaked with red or purple spots and lines.[72]

**Poultice:** Boil carrots until soft or grate if using raw carrots. Mash into a pulp, adding some vegetable oil, or mix in manuka honey for additional antiseptic properties. Spread on a cloth and apply to the skin. Ideal for infected wounds, skin ulcers, abscesses, cysts, boils, and even cold sores.

**Infusion:** one ounce carrot root to one pint of boiling water.

**Juice:** one to two glasses daily or ten to twelve grated carrots.

**Infusion of Carrot seeds:** one teaspoon of bruised seeds per cup of water and prepare as an infusion.

Wild carrot roots can be used in the first year as a food, and the leaves may be added to salads.

**Cautions:** Wild carrot seed is contraindicated in pregnancy. Extended contact with wild carrot leaves may cause blisters and dermatitis in those with sensitive skin.

Moderation is the key. Consuming too many carrots on a daily basis may lead to an orange yellowish (temporary) discoloration on palms of the hand and soles of the feet. This is a condition called carotenemia. It is a sign of ingesting too many carrots and leads to a subsequent excessive intake of carotene. This is seldom serious but is definitely a sign to decrease consumption. Consensus is that after backing off on the amounts consumed, the discoloration should disappear in a couple of days.

## Parsley Leaf, Herb, and Root

Parsley is a recognized food world-wide. Adding a delicious green flavor to foods, it is also considered an herbal medicine. There are many species. Italian parsley, common parsley, and rock parsley are all effective. The leaf is harvested in the summer months and used as a garnish in cooking. The root is used in fall. The whole plant's herb (leaves and stem), root, and seed are used medicinally. The root is considered an edible root vegetable and a liver tonic herb.

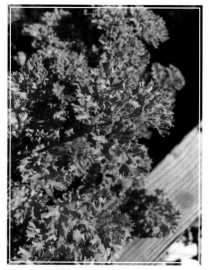

**Parsley Leaf, Herb, and Root (*Petroselinum crispum*) Family: *Apiaceae***

**Chemical Constituents:** volatile oil (apiol, myristicin, eugenol, thujene, pinene), vitamins C, E, flavonoids (apigenin, luteolin), iron and folic acid, coumarins[73]

**Medicinal Actions:** diuretic, blood purifier, digestive tonic, galactagogue, emmenagogue, carminative, antiseptic, expectorant, anti-inflammatory

**Applications:** infusion, food, juiced, topical application, hair rinse

Parsley leaf is a chlorophyll-rich, nutritious food, remineralizing to the body. 100 g of fresh parsley leaf contains 138 mg Calcium, 6.2 mg Iron, 50 mg Magnesium, 1.07 mg Zinc, 133 mg Vitamin C, 8424 IU Vitamin A, and 1640 ug Vitamin K.[74] Parsley is a rich source of calcium and also contains trace amounts of zinc and boron, both of which assist in the metabolism and absorption of calcium.[75] Parsley is an ideal green food addition to a diet with iron deficiency when the leaf is eaten raw, sprinkled over vegetables, in stews, or blended into your favorite mixed greens.

As a spring tonic, parsley is cleansing and assists removal of waste matter and uric acid out of the body. It is supportive to the liver and kidneys. Reach for its nutritious properties for arthritis, gout, and joint stiffness, and to provide essential nutrients and minerals for healthy hair and strong nails.

Parsley's diuretic effect is attributed to the flavonoid content and the volatile oils, myristicin and apiole, which are of benefit for swollen ankles, for fluid retention related to premenstrual syndrome, and any condition relating to lack of urine flow. The whole plant can be used to encourage the release of fluid from body tissues, although the seed may be most effective.

It is considered a dose-dependent emmenagogue (an agent that regulates and promotes or brings on menstruation). Apiol, one of the numerous volatile oils, is responsible for this action. For this reason, do not use during pregnancy. After birth, however, reach for parsley to offer assistance with returning the uterus to its previous measurement and proportion. In addition, parsley poultices may assist with tender engorged breasts and assist in drying up milk once breast-feeding has ended.[76]

- **For skin infections:** prepare as an antiseptic topical application.
- **For head lice:** juice fresh parsley and use as a hair rinse.
- **For gas, bloating, and indigestion:** prepare a carminative tea.
- **For natural breath freshening properties:** munch on leaves after eating.
- **As a natural deodorant:** consume the fresh leaves and prepare tea.

**Mindfulness:** When ingested as a flavoring, garnish, in normal food dosages, and medicine as directed, parsley is very safe, but do not consume parsley in large amounts while pregnant. Avoid using its root, seed, or essential oil entirely during pregnancy. Also, do not use when experiencing painful menstruation or in cases of disturbed kidney function.

# Parsley Fluid Retention Tea

**Ingredients**
1 teaspoon Parsley leaf
1 teaspoon Corn silk or stigmas
1 teaspoon Dandelion leaf

**Directions**
Prepare as an infusion for 3 cups of water. Steep 15 minutes and consume throughout the day. Do not use if pregnant or if experiencing kidney disease—it is too stimulating for tired kidneys.

## Caraway

A common spice used in East Indian curries, the seeds can be chewed to freshen breath and to promote digestion after a large meal, and also can be used medicinally.

**Constituents:** volatile oils (carvone, limonene, pinene, thujone), flavonoids,[77] terpenens, coumarins, phenolic acids.[78] One tablespoon (6.7 gr) of Caraway seed delivers 46 mg of Calcium, 17 mg of Magnesium, 91 mg Potassium, and 24 IU Vitamin A.[79]

**Medicinal Actions:** carminative, warming circulatory herb, antibacterial, antiviral, antifungal, galactagogue, expectorant

**Applications:** infusion, poultice, tincture, bath, essential oil, fomentation, syrup, honey, vinegar, and a spice in foods

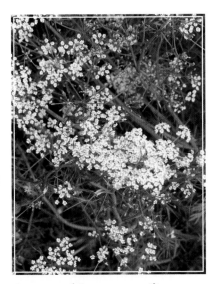

**Caraway (*Carum carvi*)**
**Family: *Apiaceae***

Caraway has been used for centuries to improve the appetite and support digestive capacities, while reducing gas and bloating. It can be prepared for an infant to reduce colic and included in mom's foods, as a spice, to reduce digestive cramping. Consider preparing a tea and bathing an infant for colic and digestive calming effects.

To assist with a spastic cough and for bronchitis, add into expectorant, lung tonic tea blends as a flavor enhancer and for its slight antiseptic and antispasmodic properties.

**Lactation stimulant:** Use caraway as a spice added into mother's meals and as an infused tea to assist with the production of breast milk. Be liberal—aim for two to four grams of tea daily for this support.

Colic is a common discomfort experienced in infants (up to 3 months) due to excessive amounts of trapped air in the intestines caused by chronic air swallowing, an alkaline body, emotional upsets, an excess of ingested sodium or sulfur, overfeeding, and/or spasms generated from specific foods that a breast-feeding mother may be consuming. **Foods to be mindful of include: milk, garlic, the cabbage family, too many fruits (high sugar), and beans (due to the fiber content). Eliminate trigger foods until the condition clears. Prepared formulas made from cows may contain additives including fructose and corn syrup, which may upset the stomach, worsening colic symptoms.

# CARAWAY ANTI-CRAMPING TENDER TUMMY RELIEF

**Ingredients**
1 part Fennel seeds
½ part Ginger root
1 part Chamomile flowers
1 part Caraway seed

**Directions**
Prepare an infusion of this tea and use as bathing water for an infant, or soak a towel in the infusion and wring it out. Apply lukewarm to the stomach (testing the heat first to prevent burning) or administer with a syringe for oral dosages. Refer to infant dosages on Page 40. For adults, drink as a tea or apply as a fomentation.

### Garlic Bulb

My enthusiasm for other cultures includes a fascination with the names of herbs in other languages. Garlic is known as *aglio* in Italian, *ail* in French, and *ajo* (pronounced as A HO) in Spanish.

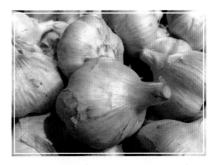

**Garlic Bulb (*Allium sativum*)**
**Family: *Alliaceae***

Harvest garlic cloves first in early spring and dig up the bulbs in the early fall to store for winter use.

Are you one who avoids garlic due to bad breath? Then consider munching on fennel seeds or parsley afterwards to minimize garlic breath, or as herbalist Terry Willard suggests, using mint-flavored liquid chlorophyll or freshly-juiced wheatgrass may freshen the breath.[80] To maximize its effectiveness for long-term conditions, consume a daily dosage.

**Constituents:** volatile oils, (alliin, a sulfur compound that is converted to allicin), B vitamins, enzymes, allinase, flavonoids, and minerals[81]

**Medicinal Actions:** antibacterial, antiviral, antifungal, cardiovascular benefits, diaphoretic, expectorant, hypotensive, antidiabetic

**Applications:** food, infused oil, tincture, topical poultice

Consider garlic as beneficial for any stagnant or toxic condition of the digestive system. A sulphur-rich food that assists liver function, it can be used for food poisoning, as an antiseptic for unhealthy gut flora, and for infections, including worms, cholera, and other opportunistic fungal ingestions such as candida.

Ingesting garlic can be an important component in a holistic protocol for dealing with any immune system dysfunction. This includes deviations in immune system functioning such as cancerous conditions; however, consult your holistic health-care provider for specific guidance.

If you are suffering from seasonal allergies, then be sure to incorporate fresh, local, organic garlic into your daily nutrition. Garlic is an anticatarrhal herb, ideal for sinus congestion and upper respiratory tract congestion in cases of allergies, and is considered an antihistamine herb. Use it with nettles and goldenrod during allergy season. In additional to clearing sinuses, garlic's antiseptic properties help to sterilize the respiratory tract. Alliin breaks down into allicin and other sulfur compounds exhibiting strong antimicrobial properties. Remember to use garlic for bronchitis, whooping cough, asthma, and recurrent colds.

Here is a fun experiment to try with children to provide a useful visual of the antiseptic actions of volatile oils. Try rubbing a garlic clove on the arch of your feet; within thirty to forty minutes you should notice garlic breath. The volatile oils are absorbed into the bloodstream and are excreted by the lungs. During excretion the antimicrobial properties disinfect the lungs during excretion, thus providing relief for bronchial infections, asthma, hay fever, coughs and sore throat. Antibiotic effects are attributed to the allicin and shown in vitro to be active against *candida, trichomonas, staph, E. coli, salmonella*, and *shigella*.[82] In addition, garlic is an ideal home remedy for those very common pinworms and threadworms in children. A traditional home remedy conducted at the time of the full moon, when the worms are thought to lay their eggs, is to consume garlic for three days and then sit the child in a bath of warm milk. The worms will exit the body, choosing the milk rather than the high-sulfur, antiseptic nature of the garlic.

Garlic is used topically to prevent infections such as gangrene and fungal infections of the feet or skin. Apply sliced garlic over a sliver, secure in place, and let sit overnight to remove embedded foreign agents from the skin.

A staple in the Mediterranean diet, ingestion of fresh garlic can be used as a cardiovascular tonic for high blood pressure, elevated cholesterol, and poor circulation. It can even help lower the risk of heart disease. It is an important addition to the diets of individuals with varicose veins, elevated cholesterol, arteriosclerosis, and high blood pressure. Studies show garlic to be a natural blood thinner, thus helpful in preventing blood clots in the body. Consider it a useful addition for cardiovascular health, for its involvement in reducing platelet clumping and raising the HDL (healthy cholesterol).[83]

When using it as a seasoning or food, use common sense. Unless one is preparing a garlicky sauce, it is unnecessary to use more than three to four cloves daily. A clove of garlic can be peeled, crushed, and consumed for its medicinal properties. Three cloves daily, or its comparison, would be the standard daily adult dose of garlic.

**Fresh garlic juice:** Two to four ml of fresh juice[84] can be mixed with vegetable juice, water, honey, or blended into apple cider vinegar and sipped as a traditional immune system enhancer or cold and flu deterrent. Some additional care is needed for individuals who are on blood thinners or statin medications for cardiovascular issues and want to use herbal medicines. The problem is not with the herbs themselves, but that the medications are so potent, they have the potential to react with many agents. In the circumstance of garlic, it may potentiate (or make stronger) many anticoagulant medications. On the flip side, consider that with appropriate clinic monitoring and guidance, it could be possible that a lower dose of pharmaceutical medication is needed—and this serves everyone.

**Authentic Alio**
3–4 tablespoons Olive Oil
3 large Garlic cloves, peeled and finely sliced
1 cup fresh Parsley, chopped
1 small, ripe Tomato, finely chopped (or a small tablespoon of tomato paste)
1 tablespoon Capers, squeezed dry and chopped
1 tablespoon Black olives, chopped
3 Green Onions, chopped
1 vegetable Bouillon cube

Start by heating oil in a pan and sautéing the garlic, onions, and parsley briefly. Add the olives, capers, tomato, and bouillon cube; continue to cook on a low heat. If you are making pasta and using this as a sauce, transfer some of the boiling water from the pasta into the sauce.

### Onion Bulb

Onions have a long history of traditional use, with loads of folklore and application. During the time of the plague, onions were hung on the doors of European homes. Inside, onions were cut and placed in a bowl in the room where one was sick. It was thought that a virus would be absorbed into the onion and not the person sick in the room. This antiseptic application may be useful as part of a larger

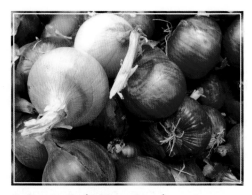

**Onion Bulb (*Allium cepa*)**
**Family: *Alliaceae***

protocol for those with strep throat and those suffering from a cold. For this reason, onions are best ingested immediately after peeling rather than hours later. Onions can grow both in the wild and in cultivated gardens. Varieties of onion vary in taste and flavor from sweet to bitter. The onion bulb is used medicinally.

**Constituents:** volatile oils, sulfur compounds (allicin, alliin), flavonoids (quercetin), phenolic acids, sterols, carbohydrates.[85] Its healing constituents contain various sulphides including allyl propyl disulphide. The constituents allicin and allyl aldehide contribute to the antibiotic and antibacterial properties. 100 g of Onion contain 23 mg of Calcium, 10 mg of Iron, 146 mg of Potassium, 7.4 mg of Vitamin C, 19 ug of Folate, and 1.7 grams of dietary Fiber.[86]

**Medicinal Actions:** Expectorant, diuretic, antispasmodic, carminative, antibiotic, antibacterial, anti-inflammatory, and repair of injured skin. Enzymes are activated upon slicing the onion, and some nutrients are lost during heating, so use raw or lightly cooked.

**Applications:** food, syrup, poultice, juice, ear drops, honey, vinegar

Onions are strengthening to the heart and beneficial as part of a larger health program for cardiovascular health. From blood pressure regulating to assisting with elevated cholesterol, onions offer optimal support.

According to *Potter's New Cyclopaedia of Botanical Drugs and Preparations*, the Allicin and alliin inhibit platelet clumping, thus offering blood thinner's effects.

The volatile oils in onion are antibacterial, antifungal, and help to clear infection. Use for the immune and respiratory tract to expectorate thick, copious mucous from the lungs. The antihistamine properties offer relief from allergies and congestion and help to clear and disinfect the sinuses. The presence of quercetin in onions assists with minimizing the body's production of histamine and increasing the immune system's resistance to pathogens and allergens. Onions are used for conditions associated with a cold such as whooping cough, strep throat, a fever, runny nose, even asthma and allergies.

I first heard of this recipe from my herbal colleague Bob McCandless, an experienced herbalist and student of the late Dr. Christopher (a medical doctor who became an advocate for the use of herbal medicine during his career). Bob would often speak of the effectiveness of onion syrup, an invaluable anti-inflammatory recipe for calming a spastic cough and for symptoms of bronchitis and asthma.

## Dr. Christopher's Traditional Onion Cough Syrup

Slice one large onion into rings. Put into a bowl. Cover completely with pure honey. Cover.

Let stand overnight. In the morning, take one teaspoon of the syrup on a spoon four to five times daily or as needed for a cough. The syrup offers antihistamine, antiseptic and antiviral properties of value for coughs, colds, and asthma and breathing difficulties, including pneumonia.

**Option:** To strain or not to strain? It is not necessary to strain this mixture. Instead, it can also be used as a seasoning drizzled over mashed potatoes, vegetables, or rice.

- **For athlete's foot:** apply fresh juice of an onion on areas of infection daily until cleared.
- **To minimize calluses:** mix half of a chopped onion and enough apple cider vinegar to moisten. Sit covered overnight. Apply twice daily. Every morning remove the layers of callus.
- **For warts:** slice onion or apply the fresh juice mixed with salt and apply.
- **To stimulate hair growth:** juice an onion and rub into the scalp.
- **For burn and blister prevention:** grate raw onion, wrap on burns to halt pain and to prevent blisters and scarring.
- **For dark liver spots on the skin:** prepare fresh onion juice applications at night. Rinse off in the morning.
- **As eardrops:** apply juice of a fresh onion as eardrops for ringing and pain.
- **For symptoms of a cold and infections:** cut an onion in half and place in each room at night to sterilize and breathe in the volatile oils while sleeping. Discard in the morning.
- **As an insect repellant:** rub onion juice on the skin.
- **For hemorrhoids**—a well-known traditional recipe: use green onions heated and mixed with coconut oil and beeswax to create a salve. Apply topically.

## Decongestant Ginger Root and Green Onion Warming Tea

4 tablespoons fresh Ginger root, grated
6–8 Green Onions, chopped
3–4 cups Water

Add the ginger and green onion to boiling water. Simmer with the lid on. After ten minutes, remove from the stove, raise the lid, and inhale the volatile oils from the steam for a couple of minutes (being mindful not to burn from the hot steam). You will immediately appreciate the natural decongestant properties from the volatile oils. Once the steam and water has cooled, drink as a tea, consuming the ginger and green onions. This is a well-known traditional remedy to use at the onset of a cold and flu, or for general congestion. I like to use this as a broth, mixing in a small amount of miso paste and drinking as a soup.

## Wound Healing and Analgesic

Prepare an onion poultice for muscle pain, bruising, arthritis, inflammations, sprains, gout, ulcers, abscesses, and for healing injured skin. Remember that onion poultices reduce swelling, and promote lymphatic drainage.

## Healing Onion Poultice

From bronchitis to earaches and infection, the sulfur rich nature of onions provides relief. Use a cotton cloth, or a towel of ample size to cover the area. Finely mince the onions; heat them or have fun sautéing as part of a meal and set aside half for a poultice. Do not heat until blackened, only until soft. Spread inside of a cloth, and fold the cloth closed. The poultice should be warm; test first to ensure it does not burn the skin. Then place on the body. Apply heat or a hot water bottle on top for thirty to forty minutes before removing. **Onion poultices are strong. Prior to application, protect the delicate skin with a layer of oil—olive oil works well—to prevent blistering.

## Onion Earache Relief

Onions have antiseptic properties to clear infections and minimize the aching associated with middle ear conditions. Roast a whole onion in an oven, cool until warm, and then slice in half. Carefully peel the outer skin and test to ensure the onion will not burn the skin. Then bind the warm onion to the ear. Sleep with the onion on overnight.

**Note:** Raw onion is too strong for the delicate skin around the ear, so roasted is best!

## Turmeric Root

With over four thousand years of medicinal use, the turmeric rhizome is a well-respected medicine in many cultures and healing traditions, including Ayurveda and Traditional Chinese Medicine. The meaning of the Latin name for turmeric comes from the words *terra merita,* referring to the color of turmeric powder as an earth-colored pigment. It is called "yellow root" in many languages.[87]

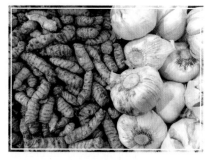

**Turmeric Root (*Curcuma longa*) Family: *Zingiberaceae***

Referenced from the book *Herbal Medicine: Biomolecular and Clinical Aspects* by Prasad, the turmeric rhizome contains a number of constituents. These include volatile oils (turmerones, also zingiberene, and sesquiterpenes) and antioxidants and color contributing, ant-inflammatory agents called curcuminoids (curcumin, demethoxycurcumin, methoxycurcumin, and dihydrocurcumin). Some of the chemicals thought to be responsible for the aroma of turmeric are turmerone, arturmerone, and zingiberene.[88,89] Rhizome is composed of carbohydrates, protein, minerals, essential oil, alkaloids, and resin.

Turmeric has a long list of medicinal actions. It is known as an antioxidant, anti-inflammatory, antiarthritic, antiatherosclerotic, antidepressant, antiaging, antidiabetic, antimicrobial, wound healing, memory-enhancing,[90] analgesic, immunoregulator, hepatoprotective, antibacterial, anticancer, antiparasitic, skin tonic, cognitive function support, digestive aid, and carminative agent.

**Applications:** Turmeric can be used chopped fresh or as a dried rhizome powder. Popular methods of ingestion include tea infusion, infused oil, tincture, in capsule form, paste, and as a spice condiment. It is also delicious added into milk, known as golden milk. Topical applications include use as an ointment, lotion, cream, poultice, wash, mask, and infused oil.

Many health-care professionals believe that chronic inflammation is the culprit behind many disease states. Thus, by addressing systemic inflammation, one can improve many health conditions. One of the constituents, curcumin, is thought to be a major contributor to the anti-inflammatory effects of turmeric. Although, using the rhizome in its whole form ensures benefit from all of the constituents, as Mother Nature intended. Curcumin provides anti-inflammatory effects by inhibiting the formation of prostaglandins through regulating inflammatory cytokines, growth factors, and enzymes, and helps stabilize cell membranes damaged by inflammation. As a holistic alternative to NSAIDs, turmeric both supports the liver and provides anti-inflammatory properties to both the digestive system and to joint pain management without side effects like gastric bleeding and ulceration of NSAIDs.

Use turmeric both internally and externally as an anti-inflammatory for acute and chronic conditions[91] such as: tendonitis, sprains, arthritis, gout, and both osteo and rheumatoid arthritis.[92] Menstrual pain and cramping can also be addressed. It is understood that the curcumin inhibits arachidonic acid metabolism.[93]

To reduce inflammation and prevent infection, reach for turmeric for skin rashes, to assist with psoriasis,[94,95] eczema, ringworm, parasitic skin conditions (such as tinea), dry skin, burns, wound healing, and acne.[96]

Known as a powerful COX-2 inhibitor, curcumin may block or suppress COX-2 pathways.[97] (Note COX-2 enzymes may activate carcinogens and assist with the growth of new blood vessels.)

Research suggests that turmeric and curcumin may offer anticancer or cancer preventive properties through antioxidant and anti-inflammatory properties, inhibiting nitrosamine formation, and through increasing glutathione S-transferase and liver detoxification enzymes.[98] Its potent antioxidant effects help prevent damage to cells from free radicals by maintaining the integrity of healthy cells, inhibiting angiogenesis[99] (limiting the formation of new blood vessels that tumors use to feed and grow in the body) and apoptosis[100] (programmed cell death). Further, curcumin may inhibit the enzyme topoisomerase,[101] which is involved in cancer cell replication. While this is valuable information, it is intended for educational purposes only; please do not use this information to self-treat. I do urge anyone who is dealing with cancer to seek out the clinical care of a health-care professional who is trained to administer herbal medicines.

As a digestive tonic, turmeric is outstanding. It has a long history of use as a stomachic for heartburn, gas and bloating, poor appetite, and diarrhea. Its anti-inflammatory nature makes this herb an ideal choice for bowel disorders such as ulcers, celiac disease, ulcerative colitis and Crohn's,[102,103] and may offer protective properties for colon cancer.[104] This herb also supports liver function, offering protection from a fatty liver. Also, its antiviral properties can offer support for jaundice, cirrhosis, and hepatitis. One of my long-term mentors, herbalist Chanchal Cabrera explains its actions as being "powerfully antioxidant to the liver and cell membranes . . . and a hepatic protective and rejuvenator akin to milk thistle or artichoke."[105] Its antioxidant properties offer liver protection from cellular DNA damage, pollution, environmental and chemical-induced toxins such as aflatoxins and cigarette smoke, assisting their removal from the body by raising the glutathione levels and promoting phase II liver detoxification.

More recent research conducted on mice has indicated that the natural anti-oxidant properties of turmeric may be of value for preventing toxicity from the well-known nerve excitotoxin, synthetic fluoride, which contributes to neuron damage and cell death during the oxidation of cellular DNA, lipids, and protein. Turmeric can help prevent cellular damage, increase glutathione levels and offer neuroprotective properties.[106] Synthetic flouride is a chemical added into our water supplies, an ingredient in certain pesticides, pharmaceuticals (including Cipro, a potent antibiotic), Teflon pans, mechanically-deboned chicken, and (the obvious) toothpaste, mouthwash, and processed beverages.[107]

- **For dandruff:** massage turmeric-infused oil into the scalp nightly; wash out in the morning.
- **To cool a sunburn:** combine aloe vera gel with turmeric powder or turmeric-infused oil and apply to the skin.
- **For swimmer's ear:** prepare a traditional ear oil (on page 238) and mix in two tablespoons turmeric-infused oil. Apply as ear drops.
- **For sprains:** mix turmeric powder with salt and fresh lime juice until moistened. Then wrap inflamed joints.
- **For relief of a head cold:** with body aches associated with a cold or flu, add turmeric into an antiseptic tea along with yarrow, peppermint, and ginger.
- **For psoriasis:** a topical application of turmeric to help reduce scaling, itching, and inflammation.
- **As an application for insect bites:** apply the paste directly to the bites for immediate relief.
- **For relief of a toothache and healing for mouth ulcers:** turmeric was traditionally used for symptoms of a toothache. As a mouth rinse, it can offer protection from mouth ulcers frequently experienced during chemotherapy.
- **For ringworm, tinea, and other skin infections:** mix turmeric powder with honey and add a couple drops of tea tree oil or the antiseptic Neem essential oil and apply as a paste.

Fresh turmeric has a stronger flavor and slightly more bitter notes than the dried. Place the powder into a spice container and leave it on the kitchen table for daily support. Sprinkle turmeric over foods such as eggs, casseroles, curry dishes, and roast vegetables. Or add it into tea or hot milk (or a nondairy drink!) using a generous application of black pepper to accompany, when possible. Turmeric paste can also be made up in advance and added to oil for cooking, warm drinks, or foods.

Turmeric is certainly Mother Nature's anti-inflammatory support for humans and pets alike. Consider adding half a teaspoon to a full teaspoon of turmeric powder daily into an elderly pet's soft food for anti-inflammatory support.

**Absorption Dilemma:** Turmeric is difficult to absorb on its own, therefore it is often used together with circulatory support herbs such as black pepper or ginger. Or it is mixed into a rich fat base such as coconut oil, olive oil, whole milk, yogurt, or butter (ghee or clarified butter being the best). One of the easiest applications is to whip turmeric into butter or ghee. Due to challenges with absorption, a concentrated tincture or capsules may provide the best results.

In the text *Principles and Practices of Phytotherapy* by Kerry Bone and Simon Mills, a liquid extract dosage varies from five to fourteen ml daily, and approximately four grams of the powdered turmeric is suggested twice per day.[108] Minor gastrointestinal side effects like nausea and diarrhea have been reported from copious amounts, but using turmeric in your foods should be without effect. For individuals taking anticoagulant medication, experiencing significant hair loss, or trying to conceive, high dosages should not be given.[109]

### Turmeric Ghee

Blend in 1/3 cup turmeric powder to the same volume of butter or ghee. Or slowly melt butter on the stove, taking care not to boil, and remove from heat. Stir in turmeric. Place in a glass container and refrigerate. Use in cooking as you normally would use butter.

There are many traditional Ayurvedic golden milk recipes. Here is one with the modern addition of coconut oil for a delicious flavor.

## Golden Paste

1 cup Water
½ cup organic Turmeric rhizome powder
1 teaspoon Ginger powder
2 teaspoons Black Pepper powder
4 tablespoons virgin Coconut Oil or Olive Oil

Boil water in a pot atop the stove. Reduce heat to a low simmer and add in the turmeric, ginger, and black pepper. Cook 10 minutes, stirring regularly until it has a thick paste-like consistency. Remove from heat, add oil, and mix well. Pour into a glass jar and cool before placing the lid on. Refrigerate and store. Use up within 3 weeks. Use this paste to make "Golden Milk" below.

## Golden Milk

2 cups Milk (almond or rice milk are delicious options)
1 teaspoon Golden Paste (see above)
Black Pepper
½ teaspoon fresh Ginger, chopped or grated
⅛ teaspoon pure Vanilla (optional)
Honey or Stevia to taste (optional)
Pinch of Cinnamon or Nutmeg to taste (optional)
Lemon juice (optional)

In a pot, heat the milk until hot but not boiling. Add one teaspoon of the golden paste. Stir well, adding in black pepper and ginger, then season as desired using vanilla, honey, stevia, cinnamon, nutmeg, and even lemon juice for variety in flavor. Drink hot or cool down and use as a delicious smoothie base.

## Turmeric-Infused Oil
1 cup of pure Coconut Oil or Olive oil
Fresh Turmeric rhizome, grated or coarsely chopped to obtain
  4 tablespoons
or 3 tablespoons dried Turmeric root

Slow cooking method: Mix the dried turmeric powder with oil. Place in a slow cooker or double boiler and gently heat on the lowest temperature for 3 hours, making sure the oil does not burn. Remove from heat, cool, and bottle. I personally do not strain this oil but rather transfer it to a glass container. Shake well before use and apply topically to the joints, scalp, and skin. For skin infections, add in a couple drops of essential oil. Neem and tea tree essential oil will enhance the antiseptic activity. As turmeric can temporarily discolor the skin, test first on a small area before using on the whole body.

## Tropical Turmeric Smoothie
1 cup Coconut milk
1 teaspoon Coconut Oil
½ cup frozen Mango, Peach, or Pineapple chunks
1 ripe Banana
½ Avocado
1 tablespoon Turmeric powder
½ tablespoon Cinnamon powder
A pinch of Cardamom powder
Handful of fresh Basil
½ tablespoon fresh Ginger root

Blend in a food processor until mixed well.

## Ginger Rhizome/Root

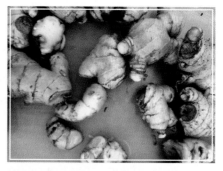

**Ginger Rhizome/Root (*Zingiber officinalis*) Family: *Zingiberaceae***

What visuals come to mind when thinking about ginger? Gingerbread cookies and those colorful gingerbread houses at Christmas? Have you ever used ginger tea or chewed on candied ginger for travel sickness? Ginger has a long history of worldwide use both as a food and a medicine. The use of the ginger rhizome has been used for centuries to aid digestion and improve blood flow to the peripheries of the body. The fresh root is most effective, as the volatile oil content is lower in dried or powdered products. The tincture and tea provide amazing medicine.

**Chemical Constituents:** volatile oils (zingiberene, camphene), resin (gingerols),[110] starch, lipids, mucilage, protein[111]

**Medicinal Actions:** carminative, digestive, expectorant, circulatory agent, antispasmodic, analgesic, expectorant, antiemetic, antiflatulent, antitussive

**Applications:** infusion, tincture, poultice, fomentation, herbal bath, essential oil, honey

Cultures far and wide have used ginger for digestive complaints. This warming, spicy carminative herb can offer almost immediate relief from indigestion related to overeating. Its antispasmodic effects can offer relief from cramping and colic. It is a great stomach settler for nausea related to car or motion sickness, and even for nausea during pregnancy (used in moderation). For antinausea support, use the equivalent of one-half teaspoon to one teaspoon of dried rhizome per cup of tea. Try mixing ginger with chamomile and fennel for an effective stomach settling aid and consider ginger chews for a fun variation.

A topical preparation is a welcome warming relief for all types of pain, including a charley horse or muscle contractions. It helps with every kind of muscle pain, including menstrual cramps, athletic stiffness, and digestive cramping. Prepare an herbal bath, poultice, or fomentation and apply over the problem area. The spicy nature of ginger is used as a circulatory stimulant for pins and needles sensation and improving poor circulation. Do you experience cold, blue-tinged hands and feet in the winter? This low-circulation condition, known as chilblains, can be reversed by simply reaching for ginger to warm up the extremities.

Ginger is also known as an expectorant herb with anti-tussive properties to calm a spastic cough. It is often combined into delicious respiratory teas for improving flavor, adding needed circulatory support, and for gently encouraging the release of mucous from the lungs for emphysema, bronchitis, colds, and respiratory infections.

For internal use for an adult, the dried rhizome can be ingested using up to one gram taken three times per day, as a tea, or used as a tincture up to three ml per day.[112] While the ingestion of ginger has had centuries of safe use for nausea during pregnancy, stay within the recommended dosages per day. If using capsules, it is suggested not to exceed ten capsules per day of standard 00-sized capsules.[113]

### Ginger Turmeric Cayenne Warming Analgesic Liniment
2 tablespoons fresh chopped Ginger root
1 tablespoon chopped Turmeric
½ teaspoon Cayenne pepper powder or ½ teaspoon Cayenne tincture
2½ cups unpasteurized organic Apple Cider Vinegar

Add chopped ginger, turmeric, and cayenne pepper to the apple cider vinegar. Pour into a glass container, secure the lid, and let sit for two weeks. Shake daily. Strain and bottle. Store in fridge. For the first use, sample on a small area of skin to test for heat and possible skin discoloration. Protect the healthy skin with a carrier oil or light barrier of cream before applying. Use topically as a warming rub, massaging into stiff arthritic joints and areas of poor circulation.

### Warming Ginger Digestive Tea
3 teaspoons Ginger root
½ teaspoon Cardamom seed
2 teaspoons Cinnamon bark
Lemon juice (optional)

Boil 2 cups of water, add in the herbs, and steep (covered) for 15 minutes. Sweeten with stevia or honey. Enjoy as a warming digestive tea and circulatory blend.

### Cayenne Pepper Fruit

Could the common name of Tabasco pepper and chili pepper be any more descriptive? The characteristic spice of cayenne is due to a constituent called capsaicin, which has been attributed with numerous analgesic properties. Cayenne peppers are harvested from a shrub with numerous varieties growing in Africa, Asia, and South America. This red spice is named after the Greek word meaning "to bite" and is related to paprika. The fruit (and the medicinal plant part) can be consumed raw (it's HOT), cooked, tinctured, or dried and powdered into a spice often used in chili or dips.

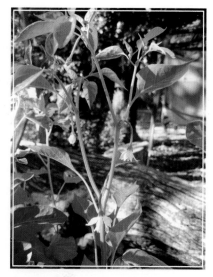

**Cayenne Pepper Fruit (*Capsicum annuum*) Family: *Solanaceae***

**Chemical Constituents:** alkaloid (capsaicin), carotenoids, steroidal saponins,[114] volatile oils, solanine, and coumarin.[115] One teaspoon of powder provides 3 mg Calcium, 749 IU Vitamins A and C, and 36 mg Potassium.[116]

**Medicinal Actions:** Cayenne is a well-known circulatory agent, cardiovascular tonic, antiseptic, antispasmodic, rubefacient, analgesic, carminative, and antiseptic. It has the unique ability to act as both a hemostatic and blood thinner. Yes, this herb does both. It coagulates blood (used for hemorrhage *and* excessive bleeding) *and* can be used to thin the blood as well! This is a plant to know, use, and respect!

**Applications:** a condiment on our food, powder, tincture, cream, salve, liniment, oil, poultice, fomentation, and emergency first aid

I learned of the virtues of using cayenne pepper years ago as a student. It has served me and many other individuals in emergency situations during the past two decades (more on this in a moment!). I was taught that cayenne pepper powder is a valuable addition to the diets of the elderly. The reason is that cayenne can be used to enhance circulation, which is often disrupted as we get older through compounding cardiovascular issues, cholesterol deposits hindering optimal blood flow, or type II diabetes, all of which reduce blood flow to the peripheries and rob otherwise healthy tissues of oxygen and nutrients. A liberal dose of cayenne powder as a condiment shaken over food will assist in regulating the blood flow and act as a gentle stimulant, ideal for those who are elderly, weak, or lacking in vital energy. It has the benefits of a heart-filled circulatory tonic, strengthening the heart and increasing the power of the pulse to send fresh blood flow to all areas of the body!

Many herbalists include a small amount of cayenne pepper in tincture blends as a circulatory stimulant to activate an herbal formula, improving delivery to all areas of the body, but the virtues of cayenne are more far-reaching than that! Many herbalists, including myself, put cayenne in the category of emergency first aid: a balancer for the heart as well as internal and external bleeding. Cayenne is an interesting circulatory *balancer*. It is an amphoteric herb that brings the body back into balance rather than creating one extreme response or another. Cayenne works as a stimulant to increase blood flow to all areas of the body, yet it acts as a hemostatic herb to arrest bleeding both internally and externally. Taken internally, cayenne can minimize internal bleeding while activating the body's "vital energy" that is essential to support life. Ironically, cayenne pepper can also be a beneficial blood thinner for daily food ingestion for those who are at risk of strokes. It can also assist to staunch bleeding. Somehow, the plant knows when and how it is most needed to bring balance. I have witnessed the effects of cayenne to stop the bleeding of open wounds numerous times. Keep this powder and a tincture of cayenne in your first aid cabinet (and your purse or glove compartment of your vehicle as well!). Reach for it for any issues related to excessive bleeding. In hemorrhaging situations, cayenne can come to our aid. Ingested internally, cayenne has protective value against stomach and duodenal ulcers, offering protection from a common side effect of certain blood thinner drugs.[117]

When using cayenne for first aid, bleeding kitchen wounds are its speciality. Cayenne powder can be sprinkled liberally (or poured into) any bleeding cut and you can literally watch the blood coagulate! I can almost predict what some readers may be thinking. "Cayenne is *hot*, it will burn!" Actually, pouring cayenne into a bleeding wound will feel a bit like a paper cut; that is certainly tolerable. And the effects are far reaching. For a hemorrhage or bleeding situation, cayenne is simply remarkable. The benefits of cayenne for bleeding and emergency situations are so numerous that it would be an asset for first responders to be taught the value of cayenne and its uses. It is potentially life saving and should be a staple in first aid treatment!

It is important to immerse cayenne directly into a bleeding wound and apply pressure, if needed. *It is ironic that in emergency conditions Mother Nature's gentle healers can be of immediate value!* Become familiar with this plant. Use cayenne in your own first aid (or kitchen cuts) and get to know the remarkable actions of this outstanding medicinal plant and then you just might remember to reach for it in more crucial situations.

These red and orange peppers are renowned throughout the world as warming, culinary spices for their circulatory effects of opening the sinuses and getting the blood flow moving to the hands and feet.

Cayenne also has other value as a topical analgesic for pain relief related to symptoms of joint and muscle pain, nerve pain, migraines, menstrual cramps, shingles, and arthritis. Its analgesic effects work by lowering substance P, thereby desensitizing nerve endings to pain. It is also a rubefacient or counterirritant, sending fresh blood flow and nutrients to a localized area. In turn, this herb is used to improve circulation, warming cold hands and feet. For those residing in cold climates, placing a sprinkle of cayenne pepper powder directly into one's socks and then heading outside into cold temperatures will encourage blood flow to the extremities and keep toes warm for longer. Remember though to wash your hands well and prevent the unfortunate action of touching your face and eyes with your hands after contact with cayenne.

Creams and salves made with cayenne can provide relief from pain, inflammation, shingles, and psoriasis.

### Some Thoughts on NSAIDs

We have all seen the advertisements suggesting the use of non-steroidal anti-inflammatory medicinal products (NSAIDs) on a daily basis to thin the blood and prevent blood clots, however these medications do come with complications. The risk of gastric bleeding and ulceration is one of the most common occurrences.

### Side effects of Aspirin and NSAIDs

In case you don't know, the use of NSAIDs are contraindicated in individuals with peptic ulcers or gastric bleeding and not recommended for individuals suffering from Inflammatory Bowel Disease (Crohn's Disease or Ulcerative Colitis). It is also not recommended for those with celiac due to similar localized inflammation, or for those with hypertension, kidney and heart disease, individuals who have undergone gastric bypass surgery, and anyone allergic to NSAIDs (for example, asthma caused by the use of aspirin).[118]

"Conservative calculations estimate that approximately 107,000 patients are hospitalized annually for nonsteroidal anti-inflammatory drug (NSAID)-related gastrointestinal complications (gastrointestinal bleeding) and at least 16,500 NSAID-related deaths occur each year among arthritis patients alone."[119]—Sourced from the American Journal of Medicine, July 1998

### Annual sales of Aspirin

According to Bayer's Annual Report, 2013, the total annual sales of Aspirin™ Cardio in 2012 reached 476 million pounds[120] and Aspirin™ (Consumer Care) reached 494 Million pounds in 2012.[121] At today's conversion rate that is a whopping $742,333,800.00 USD and $993,293,205.80 Canadian Dollar annual sales of one drug alone.

I return to considerations of safety, effectiveness, cost-friendly and sustainable, environmentally friendly, preventive health-care choices. Many herbal medicines and natural health supplements offer natural blood thinning properties, which can minimize the risk of bloot clots without the severe complications often associated with over-the-counter NSAIDs. If already taking blood-thinning medication, it is essential that you consult your health-care provider for more information and guidance. A valid possibility could be incorporating regular use of natural blood thinners into your diet to minimize the dosage of pharmaceutical medication needed. Both allopathic and herbal medicine can play a role in long-term patient care. This is a conversation to have with your health-care provider for monitoring and guidance.

This is one spice that is worthy of sitting on your dinner table in a spice container. Add a shake or two to your food daily to improve circulation and for heart health. But remember, it is a potent spice, so your body will tell you if you have taken too much. Individuals who experience heartburn or an overly sensitive stomach may notice burning in the gut. Cayenne is known as an herb that burns going in and burns going out! If you experience a burning sensation then this is a sign to reduce the dose or select a lower heat unit that is less warming. If using for emergency situations, then don't be concerned about this; the benefits outweigh the discomfort.

Be sure to wash your hands well after using cayenne in any form and avoid contact with the eyes. If you do find cayenne lingering on the skin, then use vinegar to remove, as water may not remove the heat completely. Cayenne is a rubefacient herb, meaning that it sends fresh blood and localized redness to the localized area. If using it topically in a liniment or salve, be sure to test the application on a small surface area first. A little is a lot! Cayenne is potent. Just one-third gram to one gram of powder and five to ten drops of a standard tincture taken internally three times per day is enough for circulation enhancement and quite sufficient for a daily dose! Or one can average a weekly dose at three to five ml as circulatory support.

Consuming cayenne as a kitchen spice or condiment is certainly safe. However, pregnant women should avoid taking excessive amounts of cayenne internally as a medicine unless advised by an herbal practitioner.

### Get Moving Morning Drink
¼–½ teaspoon Cayenne powder
Juice of half a fresh Lemon or Lime

Mix with a glass of room-temperature drinking water. This is the popular regime for waking up the digestive system first thing in the morning.

## Avocado Fruit

This creamy textured, well-loved, popular, delicious fruit is a food staple and medicine throughout the world, especially within South America and Mexico. It is called aguacate, ahucate and alligator pear (observe its pear-shaped alligator-like skin cover). The three main varieties of avocados come from Guatemala, the West Indies, and Mexico.[122] I would bet that most people know avocados from the delicious guacamole it provides.

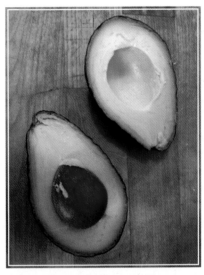

**Avocado Fruit (*Persea americana, Persea gratissima*, and others) Family: *Lauraceae***

**Constituents:** monounsaturated fatty acids, antioxidant vitamins, Vitamin C, Vitamin E, carotenoids (lutein), potassium, magnesium, gallic acid, phytosterols[123]

From the research of Dreher and Davenport, avocado is a nourishing superfood that contains many nutrients. 68 g (half a fruit) contains 4.6 g Fiber, 345 mg Potassium, 60 mcg Folate, 1.3 mg Niacin, 57 mg Phytosterols, 6.7 mg High Monounsaturated fatty acids, and 13 percent Polyunsaturated fatty acids. It also contains 345 mg Potassium, 14.3 ug Vitamin K, 1.34 mg Vitamin E (plus other tocopherols), 185 mg Lutein, 43 ug Beta-carotene, 6 mg Vitamin C, 9 mg Calcium, and 19.5 mg Magnesium.[124]

**Medicinal actions of fruit pulp:** anti-inflammatory, antioxidant, emollient, and nutritive food

**Medicinal actions of rind:** ground as an antiparasitical agent

**Applications for fruit:** nutritive food, poultice, oil, hair conditioner, cosmetic and body care ingredient in massage oils, lotions, creams, and salves

**Applications for leaf:** infusion and tincture

In Mexico, avocados have a long history of medicinal use for toothaches and gum infections. In the jungles of Peru, they are used by shamans for liver complaints.[125] The high antioxidant profile makes it ideal for use in cancer prevention. Ingesting the fruit may enhance the bioavailability of fat-soluble vitamins and phytochemicals such as carotenoids (lutein and beta-carotene),[126] which offer antioxidant benefits for eye health and anti-aging.

Avocados are rich in healthy fats that are nourishing to dry skin and used as a poultice to heal wounds. Avocado oil is finding its way into body care recipes, including creams, lotions, salves, hair treatments, and massage oils. Topically, avocado oil is applied to soothe and heal skin, for rashes such as eczema and psoriasis, and is a nourishing, hydrating moisturizer for dry skin. It assists with skin regeneration and elasticity. As a valued ingredient in hair care recipes, avocado fruit can be mashed and massaged into the scalp and hair to promote hair growth—see recipes on pages 271 and 272.

**Cardiovascular health:** Due to the high amounts of oleic acid (a type of monounsaturated fat) and alpha linolenic acid, avocados are a valued addition into one's diet for heart health and healthy lipid profiles.[127] Clinical studies on avocado and cardiovascular health indicate that dietary ingestion of the fruit can be used to reduce serum cholesterol levels[128,129,130] and can be beneficial for the maintenance of a healthy weight and metabolic syndrome.

**As a food:** This nutrient-rich fruit is used in other cultures as a baby food. Actually, it is the first solid food introduced after breast milk, and for good reason. It is similar to breast milk, with a high vitamin load and essential fatty acids. We can learn from the actions within other cultures.

Avocado oil is so nutrient-rich that it could be considered the next healthy oil to ingest after extra virgin olive oil. If you are on a dairy-free diet and love the thought of creamy smoothies in the morning, try using avocados instead. It will offer a delicious creamy solution for your recipe.

Traditionally, all parts of the avocado tree have been used medicinally. The seeds, leaves, and bark are used for dysentery and diarrhea when taken internally, or they can be applied as a poultice for a toothache. An infusion and extract contains antiviral properties against the adenovirus and herpes simplex.[131] The leaves and the bark of the plant may stimulate menstruation and act as an emmenagogue.

## Avocado Coriander Guacamole

½ small Red Onion
1 fresh red Chili Pepper, chopped and deseeded
1 clove Garlic, crushed
3 ripe Avocados
2 tablespoons Cilantro Leaves, chopped
4 ripe Cherry Tomatoes, diced
Juice of 1 Lime
Juice of 1 Lemon
1 tablespoon Extra Virgin Olive Oil
Sea Salt
Fresh ground Black Pepper
1/3 teaspoon dried Coriander seed powder or freshly ground
1/3 teaspoon or a dash of Cayenne pepper (or less depending upon your taste buds)

Chop and peel an onion, and remove the seeds from 1 chili pepper. Crush the garlic and halve the avocados, removing the seed and scooping out the fruit. Blend in a food processor until combined. Chop the cilantro leaves, and mix in the diced tomatoes. Next add the juice from the lime and the lemon, and add 1 tablespoon of olive oil. Season to taste with salt, pepper, and additional spices. Place chopped jalapeño, hummus or freshly-diced parsley around the guacamole bowl and let everyone build their own perfect dip for corn chips or rice cakes.

## Cinnamon Bark

Cinnamon is known under various names such as Ceylon cinnamon, cassia bark, Saigon cinnamon, false and true cinnamon. The distinctive, exotic scent is from the volatile oils contained in the inner bark of this evergreen tree. The bark curls upon drying, is prepared and powdered, and is made into an essential oil, or tinctured for health benefits.

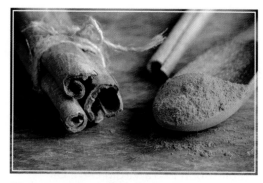

Cinnamon Bark (*Cinnamomum zeylanicum* and spp.) Family: *Lauraceae*

**Chemical Constituents:** volatile oils, tannins, courmarin,[132] mucilage, resins[133]

**Medicinal Actions:** carminative, astringent, antispasmodic, stimulant, antiseptic, emmenagogue, blood sugar balancer, diaphoretic, antidiarrheal, antimicrobial

**Applications:** infusion, tincture, powder, food, honey, spice, essential oil

Cinnamon is one of my favorite delicious warming herbs. Add it to any cold and flu recipe and think of it for cold winter days, especially when the body is chilled, and for hormonal regulation. It is a welcome ingredient for hot cereals and smoothies. Cinnamon is useful for improving circulation (so it is a valuable circulatory aid in a tea blend or a tincture formulation) and is astringing to the tissues as a tannin-containing herb. It can tighten the pores and tissues for skin care, decrease bleeding for a heavy menstrual cycle, stem internal bleeding, and aid digestion.

Include cinnamon in any digestive tea. It is delicious but may be slightly drying, effective in unfortunate cases of diarrhea. The volatile oils in cinnamon make it an ideal spice for gently supporting optimal digestion, relieving nausea and for bloating and gas. Its antiseptic properties demonstrate activity against *E. coli* and *candida*, while the carminative and antispasmodic actions are useful for colic and muscular contractions. Finally, its astringent nature assists with internal bleeding, diarrhea, and excessive menstrual bleeding during the onset of menopause or hormone conditions relating to increased menstrual flow.

Individuals concerned with elevated blood glucose and type 2 diabetes can help bring their blood sugar levels into balance by adding cinnamon powder into their daily diet. Use the powder on steel cut oats or add into smoothies. Remember to continue monitoring blood sugar levels, as daily use of cinnamon may result in decreased amounts of medication needed. Aim for 3 to 5 tablespoons of cinnamon powder per day.

If using the essential oil topically, then it is important that dilution occurs with a carrier oil, as cinnamon essential oil is an irritant. This essential oil is also not recommended for internal use.

## Cinnamon Honey

2 Cinnamon sticks, broken or chopped
2 tablespoons dried organic Rose petals
1 tablespoon Lavender petals
¼ teaspoon Cardamom seeds
500 grams Honey

Following the directions on page 230, prepare an herbal honey. Use a small amount of cardamom—it is strong. Steep for a minimum of 2 weeks prior to using. Drizzle over fruit, desserts, or use to flavor teas.

## Cinnamon Sage Ache Oil

4 tablespoons Cinnamon bark
4 tablespoons Sage leaves, dried
2 teaspoons Spearmint leaves, dried
250 ml Grape-seed Oil
3 drops Peppermint Essential Oil

Prepare an infused oil using cinnamon, sage leaves, and spearmint leaves. Heat on low for 3 hours. Strain, cool, and add in 3 drops of peppermint essential oil. Bottle in glass and use as a massage oil for athletic stiffness, sore joints, and tense muscles.

# Herbs in the Garden

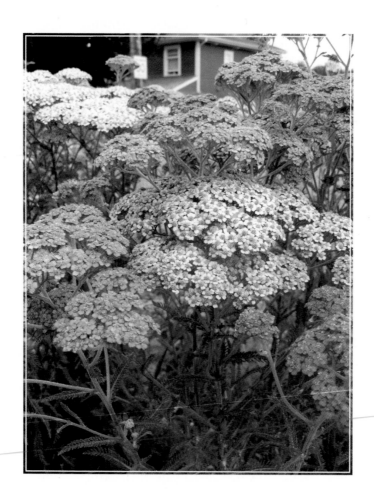

## Yarrow Flowers and Herb

Some common names of Yarrow include soldier's wort, carpenter's weed, and wound wort, offering a visual description of the medicinal possibilities of the plant. In times past, soldiers would stuff open bleeding wounds with bruised yarrow leaves to allow the astringent properties and the tannins of the plant to staunch bleeding. From summer until fall, look for yarrow's fresh flower clusters of white, yellow, or shades of pink growing along sides of cultivated land. The flowers, leaves, and stem are used medicinally, and the young spring leaves can be added into salad greens.

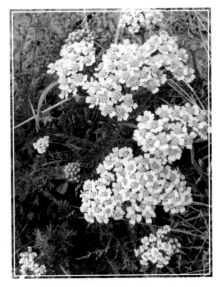

**Yarrow Flowers and Herb (*Achillea millefolium*) Family: *Asteraceae***

**Chemical Constituents:** volatile oils (azulene and chamazulene, pinenes, eugenol, thujone, salicylic acid), bitter principles: sesquiterpenoid lactones (achillin, achilleine, and many others), a bitter tonic, alkaloids (achilline), tannins, flavonoids and flavone glycosides (apigenin, quercetin, rutin), anti-platelet properties, phenolic acids, and coumarines.[134] The flavones, glycosides, and alkaloid achilline assist with the astringent process, while apigenin is antispasmodic; azulenes and salicylic acid offer anti-inflammatory properties.

**Medicinal Actions:** Yarrow is a plant of benefit for almost every organ system in the body. It is a digestive bitter and circulatory agent that is antispasmodic, anti-inflammatory, hemostatic, hypotensive, an emmenagogue, antiseptic, and diaphoretic/febrifuge.

**Applications:** infusion, poultice, fomentation, inhalation, tincture, herbal wash, essential, herbal vinegar, infused oil

To taste yarrow is to become familiar with the bitter properties in the plant. Consider the bitter actions of any plant to gently stimulate the digestive processes, improve the appetite, and encourage the movement of bile. The bitter principles, sesquiterpene lactones, activate gastric juices and support optimal digestion. Blend with fennel, caraway, chamomile and lemon balm for digestive aid.

Yarrow offers a wealth of support for the digestive and urinary tract plus marked anti-inflammatory and antispasmodic properties for both internal and external support. The antiseptic properties assist with urinary tract infections or digestive pathogens. Consider yarrow for colic, digestive cramping, and as a gentle tonic for entire digestive functions. Keep a lid on the brewed tea to prevent evaporation of the valuable volatile oils for the carminative effects.

Depending on how we look at it, yarrow can be either an efficient plant capable of many contradictory actions or balancing. As a female reproductive balancer, it can be used for amenorrhea (absent menstruation) and also for abnormal heavy bleeding, for both constipation and diarrhea.

Remember this plant for its application in colds and flus. It is a valuable antiseptic, pain reliever and diaphoretic plant. The diaphoretic effect occurs by increasing blood flow to the peripheries, opening the pores of the skin, and promoting sweating at the onset of a fever, thus lowering an elevated temperature.

Consider preparing a hot yarrow and ginger bath to soothe muscle aches, congestion, and flu-like symptoms. Place the chopped ginger root and one cup of yarrow flowers in a cotton bag and brew in the bath. For extra benefit, pour in two cups of Epsom salts and then head straight to bed—you will be amazed by how much better you will feel in the morning.

Yarrow is rich in volatile oils. Many batches of its essential oil are a pale or deep blue hue due to the varying azulene concentrations (these chemical constituents are also found in chamomile), which contribute to its antiseptic, analgesic, and anti-inflammatory properties, making it an ideal topical remedy for first aid relief of sprains, or for rashes and irritated itching skin.

Yarrow is known as a female reproductive tonic with hormone-regulating, menstrual-promoting, emmenagogue properties. It also has pain-relieving and antispasmodic properties for monthly cramping. Yarrow can be used to relieve pelvic congestion and can be combined with hormone-balancing herbs such as red raspberry and motherwort to support monthly hormonal regulation. The bitter principles contained in yarrow promote a regular menstrual cycle, and its astringent properties work to normalize heavy bleeding.

The flavonoids in yarrow offer rich connective tissue support for strengthening the walls of blood vessels and improving the health of capillaries. It is a tonic for improving general circulation, and its astringent properties create a useful agent for hemorrhoids and varicose veins (applied in a cream, infused oil, or poultice). Yarrow is also a diaphoretic plant, encouraging sweating to help reduce an elevated body temperature and thereby assisting to lower blood pressure.

**Cautions:** Yarrow is a very safe medicinal plant, but due to its emmenagogue or menstrual-regulating potential, it should be avoided during pregnancy. Individuals with excessively sensitive skin may experience itching when coming in contact with the fresh plant.

- **For hemorrhoids, vulvodynia, leukorrhea, cramping, pelvic congestion, candida infection, and wound healing:** brew an infusion and use in the bathtub as an astringent antispasmodic.
- **For toothache relief:** chew the fresh leaves.
- **As an astringent and hemostatic:** use the powder as a first aid styptic to stop bleeding.
- **As a bitter tonic for digestion and cleansing:** prepare a tincture or infusion.
- **As a natural deodorant:** traditionally, the leaves were rubbed under arms—an infusion spritzer would also work.
- **For varicose veins:** prepare an application of poultice, infused oil, or soft salve and apply to the local area.

# Hair Rinse

**Ingredients**
2 teaspoons Yarrow leaf and flowers
2 teaspoons Rosemary herb
3 cups boiling Water

**Directions**
Prepare as an infusion using herbs intended to encourage circulation to the scalp. The astringent properties may assist with preventing hair loss.

# Goddess Relief Pain Tonic

**Ingredients**
2 tablespoon Yarrow herb
1 tablespoon Red Raspberry leaf
2 tablespoon Feverfew leaf
1 tablespoon Ginger rhizome
2 tablespoons Hops rhizome
Vodka to cover (approximately 150–200 ml)

**Directions**
Use as a menstrual regulator and astringent herb for painful and irregular menstruation. Prepare as a tincture (see pages 225) and after 2 weeks, strain and use as a pain tonic. Beginning 2 days prior to menses, take a teaspoon 3 times daily as prevention and hourly as needed for pain.

# YARROW ROSE HIP COLD AND FLU RELIEF

**Ingredients**
3 tablespoons dried Yarrow flowers (or 4 tablespoons fresh, chopped)
1 teaspoon dried Spearmint leaves
1 teaspoon Licorice root
2 teaspoons dried Rose Hips
3 teaspoons fresh Ginger root
3 Clove fruits
½ teaspoon Cardamom seeds
2 Cinnamon sticks, broken
Juice of 1 fresh Lemon or Orange
6 cups Water
Cayenne powder—liberal shakes

**Directions**
Combine ingredients in a large pot to consume throughout the day. Bring
water up to a boil, then reduce to low heat and cover for 15 minutes. Strain.
Drink a cupful every 1–2 hours. Sweeten if desired. Use for children and
adults alike at the onset of a cold or flu to minimize aches and pains and to
encourage body sweating. Can assist with those under-the-weather symptoms such as head congestion, sore throat, coughing, headaches, fever,
restlessness, watery eyes, stomachaches, and general aches and pains.

## Feverfew

Feverfew grows up to three to four feet tall and welcomes the full sun. It can effectively repel insects with its bitter scent when grown in gardens. Feverfew is an independent garden plant requiring little care and attention. In traditional folklore, spring planting is said to purify the atmosphere, repel insects, and ward off disease. The large, white daisy-like flowers resemble chamomile yet can be distinguished by the leaf structure and flower center.

Feverfew's name is a play on the word "febrifuge." A descriptive for an herb with fever dispelling or diaphoretic properties, it has also been called Featherfew and Bachelor's Buttons. The aerial plant parts, leaves and flowers, are all used medicinally.

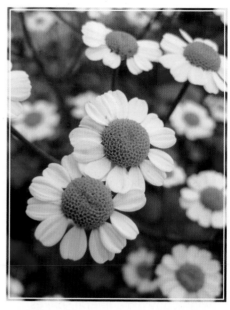

**Feverfew (*Tanacetum parthenium* and *Chrysanthemum parthenium*) Family: *Asteracea***

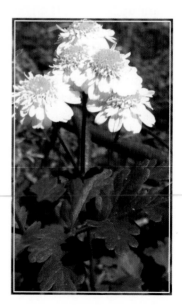

Considered a worthy female tonic herb, some have used this plant for highly emotional constitutions, low spirits, and nervousness. For menstrual cramping and to encourage the menstrual cycle (emmenagogue), begin using feverfew for pain management up to a week prior to the expected cramping.

External application of feverfew offers relief for indigestion, cramping, gas, and bloating when applied as a poultice or fomentation over the abdomen. It is also used as an analgesic for pain in other areas of the body. Place the tincture on a moistened cotton pad and dab topically, or apply crushed leaves as a spit poultice, or brew a tea in the bath to reduce the pain and swelling of insect bites.

**Constituents:** volatile oils, sesquiterpene lactones (parthenolide),[135] flavonoids, tannins,[136] melatonin found in leaf samples[137]

**Medicinal Action:** carminative, analgesic, anti-inflammatory, bitter, emmenagogue, diaphoretic, digestive, arthritis, febrifuge
(as feverfew's name implies), insect repellant, vermifuge, aperient

**Applications:** infusion (drank cold), tincture, poultice, oil, liniment, wash

Drink during a cold or flu to help break an elevated fever and encourage sweating. Or combine into a cold and flu recipe to minimize the pain of aching muscles associated with a viral infection.

This effective antispasmodic plant can be used for relieving pain and inflammation throughout the body, although its main use in North America is for migraine and headache relief. It is thought to work by inhibiting the release of inflammatory cytokines. It can also be used for digestive spasms such as colitis, irritable bowel, and menstrual cramping.

Feverfew is a unique herb in which ingestion of tea is best drank cold for pain management. Traditional antidotes ment[...]
few macerated in wine with nutmeg for nervou[...]

**Pain relief:** Prepare an infusion of the bruise[...]
cold for muscle tension and pain relief related t[...]
migraines, indigestion, arthritis, and for the pa[...]
(painful, difficult menstruation). One of the ways in which feverfew wu[...]
to alleviate menstrual cramps, and pain in general, is through decreasing inflammatory prostaglandins—agents that initiate and intensify inflammation—by "inhibiting the enzyme phospholipase A which facilitates the release of arachidonic acid."[138,139]

Although the bitter taste of the fresh leaf is not enticing to many, it is edible, and small amounts of leaves can be added to a sandwich or salad for the tonic effect of bitters to support digestion and to minimize symptoms of a headache. In fact, in a case history documented over ten months, one individual ingested three feverfew leaves every day; after ten months, her recurrent migraines subsided.[140]

## Distinguishing Between Feverfew and Chamomile

Check out the leaf structure and flower size. Feverfew flowers have white, rayed petals and a daisy-like inner yellow floret center that is nearly flat. The larger, fuller, downy-toothed leaves are thicker and alternately distributed. The strong stems ensure that the plant grows upright.

Chamomile flowers, in comparison, have a slender body and thin, fine, delicate, whisp-like leaves with pointed tips. Generally a smaller sized plant, the yellow inner center is more raised and cone-like.

### Feverfew Pain Relief Tincture

Gather fresh or dried leaves from the garden or local herb shop. Fresh is ideal if you have them growing locally. Chop finely to increase surface area for absorption and put into a glass jar. Fill with vodka—about two inches higher than the volume of fresh plants. Secure the lid tightly. Shake daily for three weeks. Strain and rebottle the tincture in a clean glass jar. Compost the herb. Use daily as prevention for headaches, migraines, and pain relief. Use fifteen to thirty drops of tincture three times daily as needed for an adult dose. Proportions should be roughly 100 g herb to 400 ml vodka.

**Cautions:** Feverfew can be a menstruation-promoting (emmenagogue) herb and therefore should be avoided during pregnancy and lactation. There have been occasional reports of individuals experiencing contact dermatitis after extended contact with fresh feverfew plant or mouth irritation from chewing the fresh leaves.[141] If you are using statins or blood thinner medication, then consult an herbal practitioner prior to using, as concurrent use with feverfew may potentiate the treatment.

## Spearmint Leaf

With so many varieties of mint, one can dive deep into discovering the various subtle flavors. All can be used interchangeably, with the whole aerial plant (stem, leaves, and flowering tops) used medicinally. Mints are harvested in the summer or spring and have square stems, slightly ridged, serrated leaves, and are generally oval or round in shape; the flowers bloom throughout the summer with white, pink, or purple flowers.

**Constituents:** volatile oil (menthol, carvone, limonene, and others), flavonoids[142]

In the case of spearmint, one of the volatile oils includes menthol, a cooling agent and local anesthetic. Recall the effects of mint flavored toothpaste in the mouth? Menthol binds to receptors, which trigger a cooling sensation, beneficial for itching and decreasing the sensation of pain. Spearmint is slightly less cooling than peppermint.

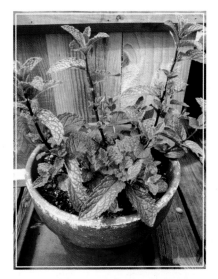

**Spearmint Leaf (*Mentha spicata* and *Mentha viridis*) Family: *Lamiaceae***

**Medicinal Actions:** diaphoretic, antispasmodic, carminative, analgesic, decongestant, anti-inflammatory, weakly antiviral, digestive tonic

**Applications:** infusion, tincture, essential oil, salves, creams, poultice, fomentation, honey, syrup, vinegar

- **As a digestive aid (for indigestion, nausea, gas, and bloating):** prepare infusion or tincture or topically apply a diluted essential oil or poultice to the abdomen.
- **For headaches:** prepare an infusion, tincture, essential oil or poultice.
- **For toothaches:** prepare a topical poultice, tincture, or infusion.
- **As a cold and flu remedy:** ingest internally as a diaphoretic and use as a steam for congested sinuses.
- **As a gentle antispasmodic and anti-cramp remedy:** use the tincture, infusion or poultice.

Spearmint gently supports the entire processes of digestion. The volatile oils in the plant are responsible for the characteristic scent of all mints and their carminative nature. It is used for settling the stomach, relaxing smooth muscles of the digestive tract, minimizing cramping, alleviating bloating and a gaseous stomach linked with overeating, colic and general acid indigestion, and settling an upset stomach related to worry and tension, nausea, and travel sickness.

All herbal tea blends created for immune system support will benefit from the addition of spearmint due to its antiviral and diaphoretic nature, encouraging sweating, and lowering an elevated fever and high temperature. The characteristic flavor is a welcome taste enhancer. It makes any medicinal tea more palatable, and the volatile oils—when inhaled—can disinfect and open the sinus passages in cases of congestion. Remember to contain the volatile oils by keeping a lid on the brewing tea until consumption.

Add spearmint tincture or a couple drops of essential oil into a lip balm for prevention from cold sores and the herpes simplex virus, or use it on an insect bite, or for itch relief from dermatitis.

Known as a cooling, analgesic herb used for athletic stiffness. Apply as a poultice, oil, massage oil, herbal wash, or in a cream for topical relief.

The essential oil of spearmint, which is not the same as the dried herb, is *much* stronger. It can provide benefit for the pain of headaches and migraines when inhaled or diluted in a carrier oil, such as almond oil or grape-seed oil, and gently applied to the temples.

**Commentary:** Now is the time to clarify the difference between essential oils (also called aromatherapy) and the use of the whole plant (tinctures, teas). Essential oils are a very concentrated distillation of only the volatile oils of a scented plant—this is what gives the characteristic scent of the plant in aromatherapy. In the case of steam distillation, steam is used to slowly break through the plant material to extract the volatile constituents. *Volatile oils are highly concentrated and need to be used with care.* Some essential oils are toxic and should never be ingested. Others are very strong and may burn the skin if applied undiluted. Mindfulness is important when using essential oils. They should always be diluted before using topically on the skin. Reach for a carrier oil such as grape-seed oil, almond, sunflower, or even olive oil—or add into a cream or salve in drop dosages. It is advisable to never consume essential oils internally unless one has had advanced aromatherapy training; some essential oils can be very toxic if ingested.

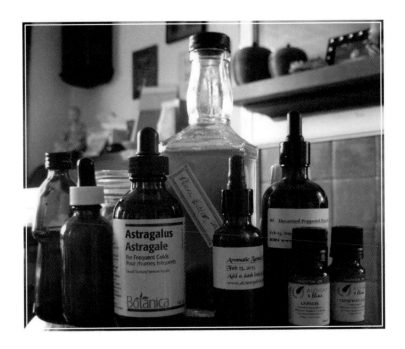

# TUMMY AND TEETHING CALM POPSICLE

## Ingredients
1 part Spearmint leaf
1 part Fennel seed
1 part Feverfew herb

## Directions
Brew equal portions as an infusion and sweeten with a little honey, or add in sliced fruit such as chopped mango or peaches. Pour into popsicle molds and freeze. These make ideal support for the pain of teething (omit the fruit and use fruit puree unless a child is eating solid food) and for a sore throat.

# Heartburn Relief

## Ingredients
1 part Spearmint leaf
1 part Fennel seed
1 part Pineapple weed
1 part organic Orange peel
1 part Hops strobiles

## Directions
Use for relief from indigestion and heartburn, a nervous stomach with gas, or for cramping and bloating. Prepare as a tea infusion using 1 heaping tablespoon tea mixture for 1½ cups of water. Steep covered for 15 minutes. Strain and drink 3 cups sipped after meals. Or for variety, prepare a larger amount and pour into popsicle molds. Freeze. Enjoy as a cold pop.

Do you purchase organic oranges? How about organic lemons? Did you know that the peel provides valuable antioxidant properties (d-limonene), which holds cancer-protective properties? Dice into small squares and gently dry on a cookie sheet on low temperature in an oven or food dehydrator. Store in a glass container and add into a pepper grinder or mix into a tea blend for added antioxidant properties. The peel of citrus fruits is a mild bitter and digestive aid. As seen in herbalist Donald Yance's invaluable book *Herbal Medicine, Healing and Cancer*, studies show that "orange peel can also lower cholesterol and dissolve gallstones. Interestingly, one side effect of many cholesterol-lowering medications is an increased risk for developing gallstones."[143]

# Vitamin C Tea

## Ingredients

2 teaspoons Spearmint leaf
2 teaspoons Rose Hip Fruits
2 teaspoons organic Orange peel, coarsely grated fresh
Juice of an organic Orange
1 teaspoon organic Lemon rind peel, coarsely grated or dried
1 teaspoon Cinnamon

## Directions

Prepare a strong infusion using 2 cups of boiling water, steep covered for 15 minutes. Before removing from heat, mix in the juice of the orange for a hot orange tea. Use herbal honey or stevia to sweeten.

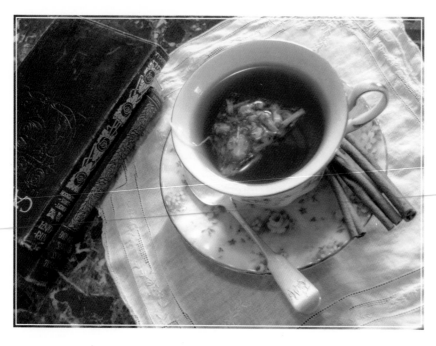

## Lemon Balm

The Greek word *melissa* refers to the honey or sweet nectar found in the flowers. Thus, lemon balm has been called "bee balm" and "the honey plant" as well as the descriptive term of "cure all." For centuries, lemon balm has been used to uplift the spirits and alleviate the blues, promoting a bright, cheerful disposition.

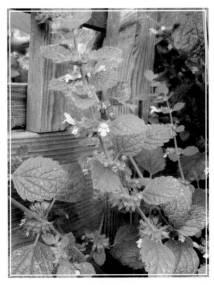

**Lemon Balm (*Melissa officinalis*)**
**Family: *Lamiaceae***

It is a perennial herb that likes full sun. For positive plant identification, notice the heart-shaped leaves, appearing opposite or at right angles to the previous leaf on a square stem. Balm is easy to grow through planting seeds or spring stem cuttings. The aerial plant parts—including its leaves, stem, and flowers—are used medicinally.

**Chemical Constituents:** volatile oils, flavonoids, polyphenols (tannins, rosmarinic acid), triterpenes,[144] bitter principles

**Medicinal Actions:** carminative, febrifuge, diaphoretic, sedative, antispasmodic, antiviral

**Applications:** infusion, essential oil, tincture, cream, oil, poultice, honey, vinegar, bath, salve, fomentation

The volatile oils can be immediately released by crushing the fresh flower or leaves with your hand (inhale the lemon scent). These constituents play a key role in the sedative properties. They have digestive-relaxing and antispasmodic effects for all digestive upsets, including a nervous stomach and associated cramping, overeating, gas, heartburn, and digestive upset. There are also benefits for painful menstruation and headaches. Lemon balm is a gentle, sedative herb to counter frequent worries, anxiety, and insomnia. It is good for sedating children who are high energy or those who are sensitive with frequent stomachaches. Traditionally, balm was used to uplift the spirits when one feels blue. Brew a tea in a bath for a young child to encourage relaxation before bed.

With its antiviral and diaphoretic properties, lemon balm is great for flu and cold symptoms. The antiviral properties are due to polyphenols filling receptor sites on cells, thus if the receptor site is filled, there is no room for the virus to attach.[145] So think of it for all types of viral infections such as Epstein-Barr virus, mononucleosis (known as the kissing disease), cold sores, and viral-related nerve pain. Apply topically to the residing phantom nerve pain after a shingles outbreak, and apply a poultice for sciatica. The more concentrated essential oil of melissa also works well topically in salves for cold sores or related herpes viruses.

Excessive ingestion of lemon balm should be avoided by those with an underactive thyroid, as "it may decrease serum and pituitary levels of Thyroid Stimulating Hormone."[146] This *does* however make an ideal herb for overactive/hyperactive thyroid conditions, reducing symptoms associated with the condition of nervousness, agitation, and generally feeling wired.

## Beam Me Up Melissa Balm Tea
1 teaspoon Lemon Balm leaves
1 teaspoon Pineapple Weed herb
1 teaspoon Lavender flowers
1 teaspoon California Poppy herb

Use as an uplifting subtle tea blend for raising the spirits and a gentle relaxant for condition of anxiety and stress. Prepare as an infusion.

## Melissa and Lavender Antiviral Shingles Infused Oil
Prepare an infused oil of Lemon Balm using dried herb according to instructions on page 233. Strain and add in 10 drops of Lavender essential oil per 100 grams of infused oil. Apply to crusted herpes sores to prevent scarring and to reduce the pain and duration of the active virus.

## Chamomile Flowers

Chamomile is an herb to know, use, and grow if you can. Consider it an important ingredient in your herbal medicine cabinet. It offers numerous gentle benefits for the whole body from digestive support, anxiety, and insomnia to pain and hormonal support.

Many species of chamomile are used interchangeably for their medicinal action, including wild, German, and Roman chamomile.

The German chamomile (also known as blue chamomile) contains higher concentrations of azulene.

Chamomile grows up to two feet in height with delicate wisp-like leaves (look for the leaves and the flower heads for accurate plant identification). Look closely at the flowers and flower center; the characteristic yellow center is surrounded by one row of white petals. Distinguish between the leaves of chamomile and pineapple weed, a shorter, smaller plant without petals (yet similar leaves). Feverfew has similar flower petals, yet with thicker, fuller leaves.

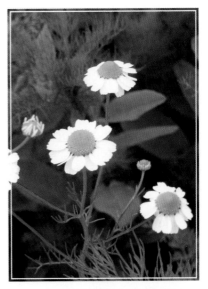

Chamomile Flowers (German Chamomile: *Matricaria chamomilla, Matricaria recutita*) or (Roman: *Anthemis nobilis/ Chamaemelum nobile*) Family: *Asteraceae*

The flower heads are used medicinally and typically harvested days after opening throughout the spring and summer, ensuring the highest concentration of chemical constituents. The taste is bitter and is coupled with an aromatic scent characteristic of the plant.

**Constituents:** volatile oils (azulene, chamazulene, and bisabolol), flavonoids (apigenin, quercetin, apiin, rutin), coumarins,[147] tannins, bitter glycosides.[148] The essential oils azulene and chamazulene both offer strong antiseptic and anti-inflammatory properties for cramping and spasms of the digestive, reproductive, and urinary tracts. It also has antiallergic effects.

**Medicinal Actions:** relaxant, carminative, antispasmodic, anticatarrhal, antimicrobial, antiseptic, digestive bitter, wound healer, anti-inflammatory

**Applications:** infusion, tincture, poultice, infused oil, fomentation, cream, salve, honey, hair rinse, salve, wash, body care, capsules

Chamomile is a traditional children's remedy for colic, anxiousness, hyperactivity, and insomnia. Many a child has been coaxed into dream time with a small dose of chamomile tea or tincture. Chamomile offers dose-dependant support for adults as well: for tension, anxiety, and insomnia. Consider preparing an herbal tea as a bath for an infant with colic and fussiness, or for a young tot with restlessness or chronic stomachache. For a loved one who is showing the effects of long-term stress and worry, prepare a strong tea and ensure it is consumed in several cupfuls throughout the day. Chamomile is a non habit-forming sedative of value for both long-term and occasional use.

## Chamomile Ginger Poultice
2 parts Chamomile flower
1 part Ginger root

Moisten with hot water and brew as a tea. Strain the liquid and apply the herbs like a poultice or fomentation. Consider a warming anti-inflammatory poultice placed over the lower abdomen for menstrual cramping. Add in freshly-grated ginger root for enhanced effects.

There is no better soothing relief for diaper rash than an infused oil of chamomile. It can be used directly for dry skin and healing, or as a vulnerary (or tissue healer) for eczema and rashes, and ulcerated or injured skin. Apply directly to the skin as a massage oil or use in a poultice or salve. Azulene offers protection from infection and is a strong anti-inflammatory.

Chamomile is *the* stomach soother for digestive upsets, worry, and tension. It provides useful support for sensitive children who have frequent worries and stomachaches related to stress. Did your grandmother ever prepare chamomile tea? It is a welcome sedative to both the nervous system and digestive system, used for ailments from a gaseous stomach, and travel sickness to indigestion and cramping. Think of it as a digestive aid. It is considered a gentle bitter used to stimulate, support, and balance the entire digestive function. The anti-inflammatory and astringent nature soothes local irritation, relaxing spasms, soothing the mucous membranes, and assisting in conditions of irritable bowel, colitis, and celiac while assisting to heal areas of ulceration. The characteristic scent of the volatile oils contributes to its carminative properties and its ability to reduce colic, gas, and bloating, soothing digestive complaints related to nerves and worry. If you steep the infusion long enough, you will be able to taste the gentle bitter effects of the plant, thereby enhancing digestion.

This daisy-like-plant has a long history as a valuable women's herb. Ideal for addressing inflammation, reach for this valuable herb for menstrual cramping, pain, and spasms related to tension and stress as well as hormone imbalance. Combine it with yarrow, cinnamon, dandelion leaf and red raspberry, for hormonal imbalance related to irregular menstrual cycles.

- **For dermatitis and dry, inflamed, injured skin:** prepare topical applications.
- **For a nervous stomach, antispasmodic, and gentle digestive:** prepare an infusion or use the tincture.
- **For teething:** let a child chew on a moistened and warm chamomile-infused 100 percent organic cotton bag when teething.
- **For hormonal-associated headaches:** use the essential oil topically or ingest an infusion or tincture.
- **For gum inflammations and oral thrush:** combine with marigold and use as a mouth rinse.
- **For symptoms of a cold or congestion:** prepare a steam or an infusion.
- **As a topical eyewash:** strain well for minor eye irritations and inflammations.
- **For symptoms of mastitis:** apply topically as a poultice.
- **For leukorrhea or candida infection:** combine with marigold or red raspberry as an infusion, place in an empty douche bulb, and use as a skin wash.

As support for seasonal allergies, the azulene constituent is thought to inhibit histamine release, preventing allergic responses while offering anti-inflammatory properties.[149] If you are not sensitive to the ragweed family, try blending this herb with nettles and goldenrod for a useful spring-time allergy treatment.

In rare cases, rashes may occur for people with sensitivities to the *Asteracea* family (including ox-eye daisy, fireweed, arnica, echinacea, and dandelion).

## Soothing Chamomile Astringent Eyewash
1 teaspoon Chamomile dried flowers
1 teaspoon Marigold dried flowers
1 teaspoon Red Raspberry dried leaf

Prepare as an infusion using distilled water. Strain very well before pouring, lukewarm, into an eyecup and bathing the eyes.

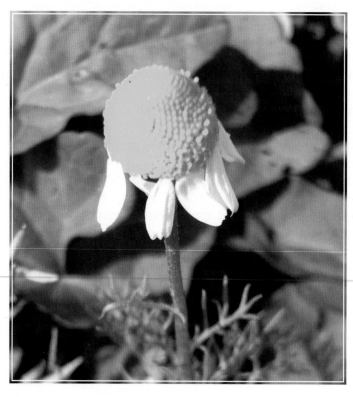

## Lavender Flowers

The origin of the word "lavender" comes from the Old French, *lavandre*, with the Latin root *lavare* meaning to wash. Historically, lavender has been used to wash laundry, imparting a fresh scent to the sudsy wash. There are over thirty-nine known species of lavender such as *Lavandula vera* and *Lavandula angustifolia,* for example, which can be used interchangeably. The leaf shape varies depending upon the species. The flowers appear as whorls on spikes, varying in color from light bluish tones to violet and dark purple.

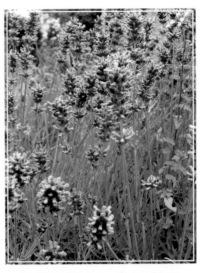

**Lavender Flowers (*Lavandula officinalis*) Family: *Lamiaceae***

**Constituents:** volatile oil, flavonoids, triterpenes, flavonoids, coumarins,[150] saponins, tannins[151]

**Medicinal Actions:** cholagogue, carminative, neuralgia, nervous system tonic, insect repellent, body care and cosmetic use

**Applications:** infusion, wash, tincture, infused oil, poultice, fomentation, honey, vinegar

Lavender's flowers are used medicinally. The aromatic scent of its flowers balances the nervous system. It is one of those herbs that help bring the body back into balance, reestablishing equilibrium. It can be used in the daytime for symptoms of uneasiness, agitation, and turbulent thoughts and as a gentle antidepressant to help brighten low spirits during intense stress and enhance feelings of calm and wellbeing. It is also known as a sedative herb, used at night for symptoms of sleeplessness, and as a carminative herb for heartburn, acid indigestion, and digestive upset.

Lavender is effective as a valuable antispasmodic for burning or shooting pain along nerves, painful joints, muscular cramping, or connective tissue discomfort. Apply herbs topically or soak in a bath with Epsom salts and lavender.

**First aid application:** The essential oil of Lavender is my favorite first aid application for burns to *prevent blistering* from scalds and burns of all kinds. The analgesic properties take the pain out of the burn while the essential oil is antiseptic. If applied frequently enough at the onset of the event, it may prevent blistering altogether.

With a recent opportunity to use the essential oil on a skin burn from hot oil, I will share the brilliant first aid capacities of this plant. For good reason the area of the burn was excruciatingly painful, red, and hot! It was a second-degree burn, extending three inches through the inside of the elbow on tender skin. To my insistence, and the doubt of the friend whose arm was in jeopardy, we applied consistent application of pure Lavender essential oil directly to the burn every ten minutes for the rest of the night, alternating with cold ice compresses. Heat radiated from the area and of course caused great discomfort. In the morning the pain was gone, and though still a hot and angry red, there was no blister. One would have expected a full blister three inches wide, considering the intensity of the burn. Reapplication of the lavender continued for day two to four. When the dead skin had lifted off of the burn, there was still no blister. By day five the redness disappeared entirely with no blister and NO visible scarring or trace that a burn had ever occurred over the area. A fellow first aid attendant had witnessed the progression during the week. "How could that be possible?" was all he said. There is really nothing more to say. Use the pure essential oil with consistency and with confidence for burns. You will be amazed with the results.

We have all heard the warning, "Don't apply an oil to a burn." Take note: don't mistake an essential oil for an oily product—it is not the same. Lavender essential oil can be safely and immediately applied straight to a burn to prevent blistering. Reach for it with confidence! There may be slight burning around the area due to the nerve and skin damage, but persevere and continue. Lavender will work wonders!

## Relaxing Balm Tincture

1 teaspoon Lavender flowers
1 teaspoon Lemon Balm leaves
1 teaspoon Californian Poppy herb

Pack into a glass container and prepare a tincture as instructed on page 225. Reach for this tincture for anxiety, tension, insomnia, occasional worries, and mild pain relief.

## Headache Be Gone

2 parts Lavender flowers
1 part Peppermint leaf
2 parts Rosemary herb

Prepare as a strong infusion using 1 heaping teaspoon of herb mixture or prepare a tincture. Drink 3–4 cups of tea daily for prevention and treatment of headaches, or take the tincture: 1 teaspoon 3 times daily.

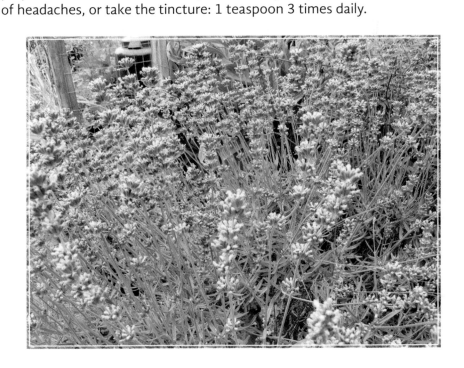

## Pineapple Weed

Known as wild chamomile (a.k.a. pineapple weed or disc mayweed), this delicate plant resembles chamomile but without petals or flower heads. It has yellowish to light green, cone-shaped flower heads but pineapple weed has no rays or petals in the center cone head. The leaves are delicate, finely dissected, fern-like, and lacy. Gently crush the herb with your fingers to release the sweet pineapple fragrance, which is characteristic of this species. Remember, wild chamomile can be used interchangeably with chamomile; they are both members of the Daisy family. This deliciously-scented herb can grow three to eight inches tall in full sun. Look for pineapple weed grow-ing near garden edges, disturbed rocky soils, and roadsides. Cut off the flower heads, stems, and leaves: they are all edible and can be used as bitter greens in salads, smoothies, prepared as a tea, or used in medicine, making it an alternative to chamomile.

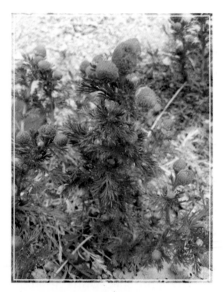

**Pineapple Weed (*Matricaria discoidea*, also listed as *Matricaria matricarioides*) The term *matricaria* refers to the womb. Family: *Asteracea***

**Constituents:** volatile oils (myrcene), cinnamic acid derivatives, couma-rins (umbelliferone), flavonoid (luteolin), diterpene, spiroethers (thought to contribute to the antispasmodic and anti-inflammatory properties)[152]

**Medicinal Actions:** bitter digestive, carminative, anti-inflammatory, anti-spasmodic, mild sedative and gentle nervine, vermifuge, menstrual tonic, insect repellant, weakly antimicrobial, antiseptic

**Applications:** food, infusion, infused oil, poultice, fomentation, tincture, wash, honey, skin wash, and body care

Pineapple weed is used as an immediate first aid treatment as a poultice (or spit poultice if out in the wild) for insect bites and stings, wounds or sore muscles. Or prepare in advance and apply as a skin wash or infused oil for an insect repellant.

A useful digestive herb, the slightly bitter nature stimulates gastric juices while the carminative and antispasmodic volatile oils are soothing for digestive upset and minor cramping, minimizing bloating and gas. The bitter components of the herb can be extracted through a longer infusion time. Prepare a tea by macerating for twenty minutes, covered. The bitter properties can be used to deter worms and parasitic infections in the digestive tract.

The antispasmodic properties make this a welcome tea or tincture of value for menstrual cramping.

The antimicrobial properties and diaphoretic nature can assist at the onset of a cold or flu and provides support for fighting infection.

## Pineapple Weed Insect Repellent
25 grams dried Pineapple Weed
10 grams dried Daisy flowers
200 ml Grape-seed Oil
4 drops Citronella Essential Oil
4 drops Lavender Essential Oil
4 drops Cedar Wood Essential Oil
10 drops of Vitamin E Oil

Prepare an infused oil as seen on page 233, using pineapple weed and daisy flowers. Strain and add in essential oils and vitamin E. Bottle. Rub into skin as needed, prior to needing insect repellant properties.

## Daisy

Daisy was once a popular medicinal herb; however, the invaluable lung tonic is not used today with the same frequency. The Latin name, *bellis*, translates to "beautiful," which is probably why the daisy is a symbol of purity and survival. Ironically, it is also considered an invasive weed; or perhaps it is one of nature's subtle reminders of perseverance. Many related plants share the common name

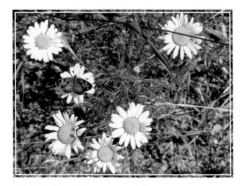

**Daisy (*Bellis perennis*)**
**Family: *Asteracea***

"daisy." It has many synonyms: common daisy, lawn daisy or English daisy, the more descriptive bruisewort, and occasionally woundwort (referring to the wound-healing properties of the plant). Both dried and fresh aerial plant parts (flower heads, stalks, and leaves) are used medicinally and can be picked between March and October.

**Constituents of flower:** organic acids; minerals; volatile oils; inulin; flavonoids—flavones, glycosides and aglycones (quercetin, apigenin, kaempferol, rutin)—tannins; malic, acetic, and oxalic acids; resin; wax[153]

**Constituents of roots:** triterpenoid saponins (primarily in the roots)

Kaempferol, one of the daisy's flavonoids, supplies antioxidant, anti-inflammatory, anti-microbial, and nerve-protective properties.

**Medicinal Actions of the whole plant:** mild astringent, demulcent, emollient, vulnerary, demulcent, antimicrobial, anticatarrhal, digestive tonic, liver and kidney tonic, antidiarrheal, anti-inflammatory, diaphoretic, febrifuge, anodyne, antispasmodic, antitussive and expectorant, antiarthritic, laxative[154]

**Applications:** herbal vinegar, infusion, poultice, skin wash, tincture, bath

Consider this plant a blood cleanser useful for skin afflictions such as eczema when taken internally with other alterative herbs, such as burdock and nettle.

The astringent nature of the plant leaves it useful for internal and external hemorrhage, inflammation of the digestive tract, and cramping. Prepare a tea and use as a mouth rinse, gargling for a sore throat and inflamed gums.

- **For mouth ulcers:** chew fresh leaves.
- **As an insect repellent:** prepare an infusion in a spray bottle and apply to the skin.
- **For a cold, flu, or cough:** use the tincture or infusion for its diaphoretic properties.
- **For headaches:** prepare a compress on the head.
- **As a digestive tonic:** the tea or tincture helps to increase the appetite and acts as a gentle bitter tonic.
- **For menorrhagia or excessive menstrual flow:** combine with other hormone balancers and astringent-rich plants.
- **As an antispasmodic:** apply topically for bruises, sprains, and symptoms of arthritis.
- **As a compress:** mix with plantain to offer support for acne and rashes.
- **For a dry cough or bronchitis:** prepare a gentle, soothing tea.
- **For wound healing, rashes, skin inflammations, bruises, swollen feet, and ulcers:** apply topically (poultice, skin wash).
- **For perineum tearing during childbirth:** prepare a poultice.

Leaves are rich in chlorophyll and high in fiber with soothing mucilage properties. Both the leaves and flowers are welcome additions to soups, salads, mixed into stews, and added into sandwiches.

Avoid during pregnancy and lactation.

## Daisy Restorative Lung Tea
2 teaspoons Daisy flower and/or leaf
½ teaspoon Thyme herb
1 teaspoon Sweet Violet herb and flower
½ teaspoon Anise seed

Boil 1 cup of water and pour over herbs. Infuse, covered for 15 minutes, strain, and drink 3 cups per day as an adult dose.

## Flow Ease Tincture

2 tablespoons Daisy flower
2 tablespoons Red Raspberry leaf
1 tablespoon Cinnamon bark
1 tablespoon Marigold flowers
2 tablespoons Yarrow leaf and flower

Prepare a tincture, following directions on page 225. Steep for 2 weeks. Strain. Use 1 teaspoon, diluted in water, 3–5 times daily to ease a heavy menstrual flow.

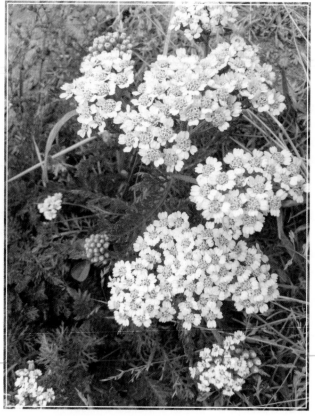

Yarrow: *Achillea millefolium*

## Sunflower

Found in open fields and along roadsides, from the southern regions of Chile and Peru all the way through Mexico and into North America, this sunny plant has earned the term "Marigold of Peru" and has the Latin name *helianthus* (derived from the Greek words *"helios"* meaning sun and *"anthos"* meaning flower). This happy plant brings a smile to those who see it. Every part of the plant can be used. Sunflowers are considered a sacred plant in many cultures. The Incas' and Aztecs' respect for this plant is found preserved in artwork around historical sites with depictions of women carrying the sunflower in their hands as an offering of gratitude to the sun gods. The entire plant (seeds, flowers, leaf, stem, and roots) has a use. The seeds and leaves are used most often in herbal medicine preparations.

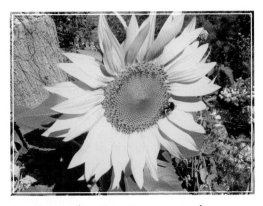

**Sunflower (*Helianthus annuus*)**
**Family: *Asteracea***

**Chemical Constituents:** The black-seeded variety of the sunflower seeds contains polyunsaturated fatty acids, making it a high-quality expressed oil and protein.[155] 100 g of dried Sunflower seeds deliver 8.6 g of dietary Fiber, 78 mg of Calcium, 5.25 mg of Iron, 325 mg of Magnesium, 645 mg of Potassium, 5 mg of Zinc, 8.33 mg of Niacin B3, 1.48 mg of Thiamine B1, 1.345 mg of B6, 227 ug Folate, 35.17 mg of Vitamin E, 18.52 g of Monounsaturated fatty acids, and 23.13 g Polyunsaturated fatty acids[156]— sunflower seeds are a superfood.

**Medicinal Actions of seeds:** diuretic, expectorant, antiseptic, antitussive, diaphoretic; used for colds, chest congestion, and as a stop-smoking aid

**Medicinal Actions of leaf:** astringent

**Applications:** infusion, food, poultice, infused oil, syrup; decoction of the seed for a demulcent cough remedy

- **For a lung tonic, elevated fever, or for expectorating congestion in the lungs:** prepare an infusion or topical poultice from the leaf and seed, or a decoction from the seed.
- **To relieve diarrhea or for a diuretic:** prepare an infusion from the leaf.

This recipe is a variation of a **Traditional Bronchitis Elixir** referenced online from Mrs. Grieve's *A Modern Herbal*.

60 grams Sunflower seeds, slightly browned/roasted
10 grams Mullein leaf and flower
15 grams Star anise or Fennel seed
¾ cup Brandy
½–¾ cup organic Cane Sugar

Boil slightly-roasted seeds in 4 cups of water and simmer down to just over 1½ cups. Ten minutes before removing from the heat, add the mullein and anise or fennel. Cover and simmer on low heat for an additional 10 minutes, then strain. Add ¾ cup of brandy and ¾ cup of organic cane sugar. Bottle. Adult dosages vary at 1–2 teaspoonfuls, three or four times a day as needed for a spastic cough.

According to Mrs. Grieve, in her well-referenced text *A Modern Herbal*, roasted sunflower seeds can also make a traditional poultice for use over the chest to treat whooping cough, bronchitis, and congestion. A tincture from the sunflower seed, taken internally, provides immeasurable benefits for treatment of malaria. This is an alternative to quinine and has high benefits for high fevers, malaise, body aches, and symptoms of shivering and sweating. A warm poultice using the sunflower leaves was traditionally mixed with warm milk. It was then used to wrap a feverish body, creating a diaphoretic, temperature-lowering effect. Historically, reapplication of the poultice was done until the fever returned to normal.[157] A poultice used by First Nations people was made with astringent leaves or the drawing root to pull out the venom of snake and insect bites. The roots were ground up and applied for healing wounds and stiff joints.

Dried sunflower seeds contain numerous nutrients. 100 g offers 78 mg Calcium, 325 mg Magnesium, 5 ml Iron, 5 mg Zinc, 35.17 mg Vitamin E, Potassium, B vitamins, and fatty acids.[158] Sunflower offers anti-inflammatory and antispasmodic properties for breathing difficulties, prevention of migraines, muscle cramps, tension, and pain in the body.

**As a valuable food:** Tightly closed young spring buds can be boiled, creating a pleasant dish served like artichoke hearts. Sunflower seeds are a familiar snack and a welcome distraction to some individuals intending to quit smoking and want something to do with their hands. Sunflower seeds can be sprouted and added to salads and sandwiches; they are delicious and perhaps my favorite of all the nutritious sprouts. In Mexico, sunflower seeds are ground up to make a porridge called *Atole de Teja*. It is frequently prepared with cinnamon sticks and a sweetener such as honey. The leaves can be used in herbal tobacco-smoking mixtures along with mullein, sage, thyme, and other herbs.

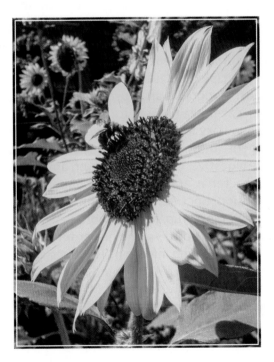

## Marigold Flowers

Newcomers to herbal medicine are often confused by the three interchangeable names, English marigold, pot marigold, and Calendula, which all refer to the same plant. Although both are in the daisy family, it is important to note that the edible medicinal calendula is *not* the same plant as French Marigold, which has a different Latin name, *Tagetes patula*, and limited medicinal use.

Reputed to be the most hearty and easy to grow flower, it is known to ward off aphids in the garden. Collect the vibrant yellow orange petals when blooming throughout the summer and use as edibles in salads or dried for numerous applications in herbal medicine.

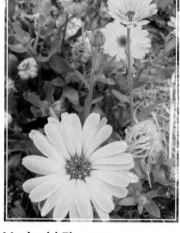

**Marigold Flowers (*Calendula officinalis*) Family: *Asteracea***

**Constituents:** volatile oils, flavonoids (quercetin, rutin), triterpenes (saponins),[159] carotenoids, bitter principles, polysaccharides[160]

**Medicinal Actions:** Marigold is an antiseptic, disinfectant, and wound healer. I always pack calendula tincture for travel as well as for a home first aid antiseptic and vulnerary for healing open cuts and wounds. It is anti-inflammatory, astringent, antimicrobial, antiseptic, cholinergic, emmenagogue, diaphoretic, digestive, hemostatic, bitter, anticatarrhal, antifungal, antispasmodic, antibacterial, anthelmintic, and immune stimulant.

**Applications:** infusion, tincture, poultice, infused oil, herb bath, poultice, cream, salve, throat gargle, syrup, fomentation, salve, spray

Think of marigold as *the* go-to wound healer for reducing inflammation and irritation and for preventing infection. The tincture or a cream is all you really need for open wounds. As a wound healer and antiseptic herb, the actions of marigold are unprecedented. Marigold helps speed up rapid epithelization of tissues,[161] stimulating skin healing and preventing infection from any open wound, scratches, and ulcers. I use this herb topically for any and all nicks in the skin instead of over-the-counter medicated creams, such as Polysporin. At my office, Alchemy & Elixir Health Group, our marigold cream is one of our bestsellers, beneficial for all types of first aid care. As an antiseptic and for speeding up the healing of wounds, it is an excellent base cream to which additional tinctures or essential oils may be added to create a custom cream.

Think of marigold as an internal and external antiseptic. Its antimicrobial properties offer value for both internal immunity as well as skin infections such as athlete's foot, abscesses, cold sores, and shingles virus.

Prepare an infused oil of marigold for cradle cap in an infant, and ever so gently massage the infused oil into the crusty, scaly areas of excess sebum. After a day or so, the crusts will dry out and separate from the scalp and can then be gently lifted off the scalp.

As a cream, poultice, herbal wash, or infused oil, marigold can be used to treat the skin of dry, cracked heels. It even reduces inflammation and ensures immediate healing for nipples that are raw from breast-feeding. For the inflammation of mastitis or for mumps or gland inflammation, prepare a poultice.

- **As an anti-inflammatory and antiseptic:** apply to swellings, sunburn, rashes, ulcers, wounds, sores as a poultice or wash.
- **For an eyewash:** prepare an infusion for eye inflammations, conjunctivitis, and seasonal allergies.
- **As a bitter digestive tonic to enhance digestion and improve liver function and bile flow:** prepare a tincture or tea.
- **To stop bleeding:** take internally and apply externally.
- **For allergies and sinus congestion:** combine with nettles, plantain, and goldenrod as a tea or tincture for antihistamine properties.
- **For athlete's foot, or stubborn toenail infection:** mix with other antiseptic herbs, such as oregano, as an antifungal footbath.
- **For varicose veins:** prepare a poultice with red raspberry.
- **For strep, tonsillitis, thrush, and sore, bleeding gums:** use a throat gargle with an infusion or tincture.
- **For antidiarrheal effects and astringent, binding properties for loose bowel movements:** use a tincture or strong infusion.
- **For candida yeast infection and leukorrhea:** prepare an infusion of calendula, thyme, and chamomile—using equal parts as a topical wash.

- **For allergies and colds:** mix together with rose hips, self-heal, and a strong infusion.
- **Hemorrhoid treatment:** prepare a poultice or cream to soothe tissues, relieve inflammation, and for antiseptic properties.

Marigold's bitter properties are of value to the digestive tract as well as the reproductive system. The bitter agents provide emmenagogue properties that regulate menstruation and provide gentle liver support. Combine as an infusion with hormone regulators such as red raspberry and yarrow to regulate a cycle, to reduce heavy bleeding, and to regulate an irregular cycle or for an absent cycle (amenorrhea).

As a digestive, marigold's bitter properties support the whole digestive function, encouraging peristalsis and assisting in healing a leaky gut. Its antiseptic and anti-inflammatory properties can be ideal for digestive ulcers and digestive infections such as candida.

Internally, marigold offers anti-inflammatory and immune-stimulant properties as well. It contains antifungal and antibacterial properties against staph and strep bacteria, and can offer protection against parasites.

### Rash B Gone Balm
50 ml Marigold infused oil
50 ml Chickweed infused oil
3 drops Lavender Essential Oil
3 drops Patchouli Essential Oil
Beeswax

Prepare infused oils according to directions on page 233. Then follow the salve-making process on page 234, taking the salve off the heat and adding in the essential oils right before pouring into containers. Makes three 50–60 ml container-sized salves. It is a great all-purpose healer for dry skin, rashes, and irritation.

## Marigold Antiseptic Tincture

Marigold flowers, dried
Vodka

Pack the marigold flowers well into a glass container (if the flowers are whole, I suggest breaking them apart so there is more surface area to come in contact with the extraction liquid). Follow the tincture-making instructions on page 225. Macerate for 3 weeks. Strain and bottle. Use this tincture topically and internally for all antiseptic needs.

## Marigold Vein Liniment

2 tablespoons dried Marigold flowers
2 tablespoons Yarrow flowers
1 tablespoon Self-heal herb
Approx. 100 ml Distilled Witch Hazel Water (available from a health food store or drug store)

This liniment is prepared exactly like a tincture, except it is intended for external use only. Mention this on the label. Pour enough witch hazel over to cover the dried herbs and macerate for 2 weeks. Strain and bottle. Keep in the fridge. Apply topically to areas of inflammation and varicose veins. The easiest application is to moisten muslin with water, cutting large enough to cover the inflamed area. Pour on the liniment and wrap the area. Provides immediate cooling relief and anti-inflammatory support to the inflamed tissues.

## Chickweed

Chickweed, one of the most common weeds, is found growing in all parts of the world. The French common name *Stellaire* refers to a constellation of the stars named after the heavens' brilliant stardust. Chickweed has also been called starweed and starwort because of its divided, tiny, white, star-shaped flower petals. It looks like ten tiny-rayed narrow petals. It is found nestled in the five green sepals surrounding the petals. One does not need to go far to find chickweed. It is likely already close by. Look around street curbs and light poles.

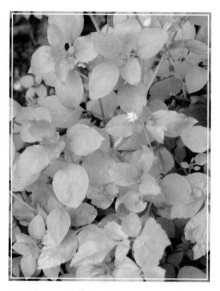

**Chickweed (*Stellaria media*)**
**Family: *Caryophyllaceae***

Look for a trailing plant with a tangled mat of delicate, lush green stems, egg-shaped leaves formed into a point and placed on the stem in equal pairs (with or without a leaf stalk depending upon the species). For positive plant identification, look even closer and notice the tiny white tufts of fine hairs running vertically up one side of the stem only.

The herb is gathered from May through July. The whole herb is used medicinally, and this delicate, tiny plant is a delicious edible green added into salads. It can be prepared fresh, steamed briefly (no more than five minutes) or dried and stored for future use. Some species are very furry, requiring brief cooking to make them more palatable.

**Constituents:** saponins, coumarins, triterpenoids, flavonoids, ascorbic acid.[162] Chickweed is a nutritional powerhouse, providing vitamins C, rutin, A, D, folic acid, riboflavin, niacin, and thiamine, as well as the minerals calcium, potassium, manganese, zinc, iron, phosphorus, sodium, copper and silica.[163]

**Medicinal Use:** refrigerant, demulcent, vulnerary, alterative, anti-itch, emollient, mild laxative, antirheumatic

**Applications:** poultice, nutritive green in salads, infusion, infused oil, salve, herbal bath, skin wash, fomentation, juiced, tincture

Chickweed is viewed by herbalists as a refrigerant, an agent used to remove excess heat from the body. Think of it for relief from inflamed and hot, itchy skin. Chickweed's cooling anti-inflammatory actions make an ideal application for hot swellings, skin ulcers, infections, abscesses, eczema, cradle cap, diaper rash, sunburns, dry skin and wound healing of all kinds. Any topical application will work, though I am fond of chickweed-infused oil, poultices, and salve for topical afflictions.

- Chickweed is a spring tonic and gentle cleanser with slight laxative properties, called a depurative or cleanser. Use the fresh juice of chickweed as a morning tonic and purifying blood cleanser for stubborn, itchy skin conditions.
- A galactogogue of benefit to increase lactation in breast-feeding mothers.
- Eye wash: prepare an infusion of chickweed for irritation and inflammation.
- Well-known Canadian herbalist and Elder Terry Willard, uses chickweed for its stomach-healing properties in circumstances where there is bleeding in the digestive tract or the lungs.[164]

### Infused Oil of Chickweed

Gently wilt fresh chickweed for 24 hours before preparing, or used dried. Fill a container with chickweed, pack down well, and chop the stalks for easier maceration. Pour on grape-seed oil or sunflower seed oil, cover with a secure lid, and let sit for 2–3 weeks. Strain and bottle.

Both of my cats are curious about chickweed. They are drawn to the small and delicate herb and its fresh green scent. If you serve soft food to your pet, consider mincing and mixing this nutritious herb in for peak nutrition. It supplies trace minerals and also protects from hair balls.

The addition of fresh chickweed will brighten any recipe. It contributes a fresh green taste to salads, sandwiches, stews, and soups; mince like chives and add on top of mashed potatoes or sauté like spinach to add into quiche, omelettes, or a side vegetable dish. Prepare delicious chickweed pesto using fresh chickweed, garlic, sunflower seeds, and olive oil with your favorite herbs as seasoning.

## Chickweed Burdock Gout Blend
2 teaspoons Chickweed herb
2 teaspoons Burdock root
3 teaspoons Nettle leaves
3 teaspoons Yarrow leaf and flower
Black Cherry concentrate

Prepare as a strong infusion, adding in some Black cherry concentrate as flavoring and to enhance the gout activities of the blend.

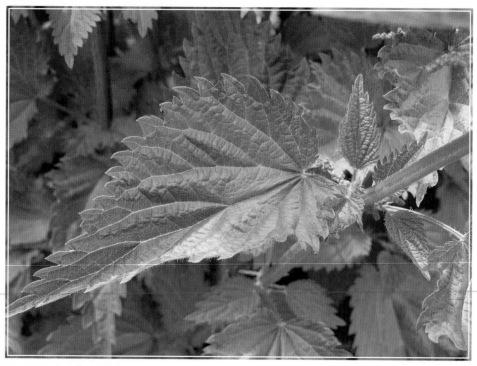

**Nettles:** *Urtica dioica*

## Plantain Leaf

Plantain is another of those valuable whole body tonics. It is used for general first aid and more. From the sinuses to the lungs, mouth, skin, digestive and urinary tracts, this herb offers healing. Where I live there are two types of plantain (*and no I am not referring to the plantain vegetable which resembles a banana). Lance leaf or ribwort plantain, *Plantago lanceolata*, and broad leaf plantain or *plantago major*. *Plantago lanceolata* has thin, long, narrow, lanced leaves. Broad leaf plantain (*Plantago major*) has fuller egg-shaped leaves with thick vein-like netting in the leaf. Both plant species can be used interchangeably. Plantain has also been called ribgrass, ribwort, rat's tail (for obvious reasons) and ripple grass.

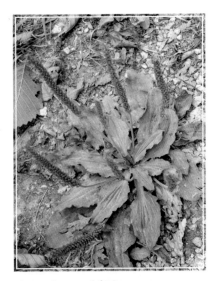

**Plantain Leaf (*Plantago lanceolata, Plantago major*)
Family: *Plantaginaceae***

The place to identify plantain is in your lawn; as it is a known lawn weed, it is also identified mingling between the grass, near paved roads, or parks. The leaf has no scent, and when chewed it is slightly mucilaginous. The leaves are used medicinally and harvested during the summer or picked at any time for emergency first aid solutions.

**Chemical Constituents:** iridoids (aucubin), flavonoids (apigenin, luteolin) allantoin, tannins, furmaric acid,[165] resin, saponins, acids (fumaric, ursolic, ascorbic acid, salicylic acid), alkaloids, mucilage[166]

**Medicinal Actions:** demulcent, astringent, antibacterial, a blood tonic, lymphatic, diuretic, anti-inflammatory, expectorant, antihistamine, anti-hemorrhagic, anticatarrhal properties

**Applications:** infusion, tincture, poultice, fomentation, liniment, salve, cream, infused oil, syrup

If you ever choose to chew on the leaf (for spit poultices below) you will notice the slightly slippery, mucilaginous properties of the leaves. These soothing properties have benefit internally to the mucous membranes of the respiratory tract, urinary and digestive systems, and are beneficial for external treatment of aches and swellings. Combine this plant with mullein for soothing persistent coughing and for bronchitis.

Plantain can be considered a daily tonic for its high nutrient content and tonifying properties on the whole body systems, particularly the mucous membranes. Nutritive tonic: an excellent source of chlorophyll and packed full of minerals, including zinc, potassium, and silicic acid.[167]

Plantain is a soothing anti-inflammatory mucous membrane tonic of benefit for urinary, diuretic, digestive, respiratory complaints that works in a number of ways. Plantain contains tannins, which help to minimize swellings. Plantain can be used for bleeding skin wounds, hemorrhoids, inflamed gums, and for symptoms of a toothache—either munch the leaves and hold in the mouth next to the toothache creating an oral poultice, or use the tea or tincture as a mouth rinse. Due to the constituent allantoin, also contained in comfrey, plantain is an ideal wound healer, good for quick cell regeneration of damaged skin.

For digestion plantain offers soothing relief for internal bleeding, gut and digestive inflammations, and diarrhea. Aucubin may offer liver protective properties.[168]

As an antihistamine and anticatarrhal herb, plantain can suppress excess secretion of mucous. Use it for sinus congestion, allergies, and bronchial congestion with copious mucous. Combine with expectorant and antiseptic herbs for breathing support and lung infections. For the urinary tract, plantain is a valued ingredient for muscle contractions, bleeding, and irritation.

Prepare an infusion and use as an eyebath for conjunctivitis and irritated eyes, or use as a skin wash for promoting healing for an open cut or insect bite.

The perfect application as a spit poultice for pulling out slivers or agents imbedded into the skin, think of plantain as nature's solution for a bug bite as well as for assisting the withdrawal of venom from insect stings and removing infection from an abscessed wound. Saliva in human mouths contains a protein called epidermal growth factor that may assist with cell proliferation.

## Soothing Plantain Cough Ease Tea

1 part Plantain leaf
½ part Thyme leaf
2 parts Mullein herb
1 part Fennel seeds
1 part organic Orange peel
*Optional—add in medicinal honey

Prepare an infusion, syrup, or tincture. Use as needed for a spastic dry cough.

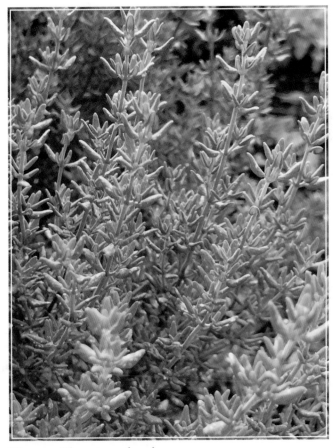

**Thyme: *Thymus vulgaris***

## Dandelion Leaf and Root

Rumored to be the world's most notorious weed, this is also a revered medicinal plant. Once rooted in a garden, it is sure to stay around; its underground root system can reach over sixty centimeters in length. When pulled up, the roots regrow from just one piece of root and another dandelion surfaces. The French word *pissenlit* refers to dandelion's efficient diuretic properties. It is also named lion's tooth for the notched shape of the leaves, resembling teeth. Medicinally, the root, leaves, and milk from the stem are used. Add the fresh flowers and leaves into salad greens. Harvest for medicine after the second year of growth; collect the roots in the early spring and pick the leaves in spring or early summer.

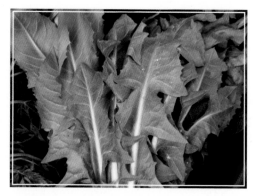

**Dandelion Leaf and Root (*Taraxacum officinalis*) Family: *Asteracea***

Have you ever observed a dandelion long enough to notice that its flowers close up in the evening and cloudy weather? This plant enjoys the sun! Have you ever tried to count the petals? The yellow flowers contain countless tiny rayed petals.

There are many dandelion look-alikes, known as false dandelion. True dandelion has angular leaves growing directly out of the base of the root crown at ground level (there are no branches, hairs, or leaves on any central stalk). The unforked, hollow stem of the plant gives off a milky white sap. Look closely at the leaves— they should not be fuzzy, spiny, or prickly. These qualities indicate another plant.

**Constituents:** sesquiterpene lactones, triterpenoids (beta-Sitosterol, taraxol), phenolic acids, carotenoids (lutein), inulin, pectin,[169] acids (linolenic acid, linoleic, oleic), potassium, vitamin A, 100 g of fresh leaf offers 14 000 IU, resin, phytosterols.[170]

**Medicinal Actions:** choleretic, antilithic, diuretic, nutritive, alterative, bitter tonic, mild laxative. A valuable cleaner and detoxifier, dandelion supports the organs of elimination. Dandelion can balance the fluids of the body and is a liver and kidney tonic.

**Applications for leaf:** infusion
**Applications for root:** decoction; tincture, vinegar, nutritive
**Nutritive tonic:** Add fresh dandelion leaves to a salad for their high iron content. 100 g of raw Dandelion leaves provides 3.5 grams of Fiber, 187 mg Calcium, 3.1 mg Iron, 36 mg Magnesium, 397 mg Potassium, 35 mg Vitamin C, 27 ug Folate, trace amounts of B Vitamins, 10 161 IU Vitamin A, 3.44 mg of Vitamin E, and 778 ug Vitamin K.[171] Use as a food to build the blood for conditions of anemia and for its high potassium content.

Dandelion is an effective cleanser for all the organs of elimination—the colon, kidneys, and liver—for all around detoxification.

Dandelion leaf might very well be considered one of the best diuretics in the natural world. Unlike pharmaceutical diuretics (when a doctor may suggest daily ingestion of a banana to replenish lost potassium levels), dandelion is already mineral-rich and packed full of potassium, replenishing minerals as it removes large amounts of fluid from the body. Drink the tea infusion for high blood pressure and relief from fluid retention related to premenstrual tension or from the effects of travelling on an airplane. The leaf encourages release of fluid from the body, eliminates uric acid buildup, and removes waste matter from the body in conditions of arthritis, gout, and other degenerative disorders.

The root is a gentle bitter; it can be decocted and used as a replacement for that morning coffee (some people enjoy roasting the root for a stronger taste and then mixing it with chicory root). The bitter properties encourage optimal digestion, providing a weak laxative effect for chronic constipation, and supporting liver function and detoxification. Dandelion root can be used for periodic seasonal cleansing, for a liver detox and jaundice. Dandelion leaf and root are ideal herbs for stubborn skin conditions, from teenage acne and congested skin to monthly menstrual breakouts, psoriasis, and itchy skin. It is also of benefit for those whose livers could use some support (either from alcohol ingestion or numerous medications).

As a women's herb, both the leaf and root are valuable. Everyone can benefit from liver support and this is often the missing ingredient for women who are experiencing a more challenging transition through menopause, as the liver is needed for breaking down excess circulating hormones and balancing hormones. Add into a tea or tincture for liver support.

Dandelion roots contain a chemical called inulin, which contains fructo-oligosaccharides (FOS), known as food for healthy gut bacteria. So consume this bitter root in teas on a weekly basis for digestive health.

- **As a coffee substitute:** prepare dandelion root coffee (roasted or raw) for digestive support and a mild laxative; use instead of coffee in the morning.
- **For those annoying plantar warts:** paint the wart faithfully with the white milky sap from dandelion stem.
- **As a diuretic:** prepare dandelion leaf as an infusion.
- **For a liver tonic:** prepare a decoction from the root—and ingest for skin conditions and liver support.

Due to dandelion root's liver-stimulating properties, and considering that the liver manufactures bile, for those with gallstones or active blockage of bile ducts, dandelion root should be avoided.

## Dandelion Root Syrup

10 grams Dandelion root
10 grams Dandelion leaf
10 grams Watercress herb
10 grams Nettle leaf
10 grams Red Raspberry leaf
15 grams seedless Rose Hip fruit
3 dried organic sulphite-free Apricots, diced finely, seeds removed
½ teaspoon Cinnamon bark
1 quart Water
½ cup Molasses

Bring water to a boil. Add in all ingredients (except molasses) and reduce heat. Simmer. Prepare a syrup as found on page 228. Reduce liquid to about ¼ (or 1 cup). Strain. Add in molasses. Bottle and store in the fridge. Use daily on the spoon or mixed into a smoothie or cereal to build the blood and for absorbable bioavailable iron.

## Self-Heal

Self-heal is another multipurpose plant offering many first aid options for its use. It easily grows in a garden and it can often be discovered growing wild, covering sunny fields with lilac, crimson, or white petals.

A member of the mint family, some common names include "heal all" and "carpenter's herb" for its wound healing ability; also called "heart of the earth" and "blue curls." The leaf and whole herb is used medicinally and collected in summer. According to herbalist Anne McIntyre, the layered petals resemble a throat with swollen glands, and today this herb is a welcome antimicrobial gargle for inflammations of the mouth and sore throat.[172]

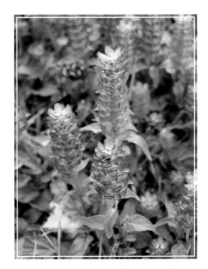

**Self-Heal (*Prunella vulgaris*)**
**Family: *Lamiaceae***

**Constituents:** antioxidants, including rosmarinic acid and triterpenes (urosolic acid),[173] volatile oil (rosmarinic acid, camphor and fenchone), bitters, saponins (urosolic acid), tannins, glycoside (aucubin), flavonoids (rutin).[174] One of the chemical constituents, urosolic acid, is an effective diuretic to help remove uric acid through the kidneys. Consider this plant for rheumatism, arthritis, and gout.[175]

**Medicinal Action:** astringent, hemostatic, vulnerary, anti-inflammatory, relaxant, antibiotic with antiviral properties, astringent, diuretic, digestive, liver tonic, antiallergenic and antioxidant

**Applications:** infusion, gargle, enema, poultice, cream, ointment, tincture, syrup

For hemorrhoids, fissures, diarrhea, and varicose veins, remember those astringent tannins to help to tighten tissues, minimize inflammation, and reduce bleeding both internally and externally; or use to reduce symptoms of a sore throat, mouth sores, and gum inflammations.

As a tea or tincture for digestive support, the tannins are of value for the toning of mucous membranes for inflammatory bowel disease, colitis, gastric bleeding, and an upset stomach.

Antiseptic with antiviral properties, it is used as a gargle for strep throat and swollen glands. It can also be considered for all other ailments of viral origin, such as cold sores, shingles, a cold, mononucleosis, glandular fever, and other lymphatic swellings.

The antioxidant[176] and immune-modulating polysaccharides provide valuable support for immune system enhancement; modern research is investigating the use of self-heal for chronic disease including chronic fatigue, allergies, and even cancer.[177,178]

Externally, self-heal is an amazing wound healer. Perhaps this is the most well-known application of the herb: a topical poultice, bath or skin wash can be used to heal open wounds, bruises, boils, mumps, and inflammatory skin eruptions. Prepare a lip balm with the tincture or infused oil of self-heal and lemon balm for cold sores. If camping or in the outdoors, the herb prepared as a spit poultice can be applied to bleeding wounds.

Prepared as a tea and used as an eyewash, self-heal can offer relief for inflammations of the eyes such as conjunctivitis, blepharitis, and styes. Add in some calendula and chamomile and you have a potent antiseptic eye rinse.

- **As an antiseptic eyewash:** prepare an infusion mixed with calendula and chamomile.
- **For insect bites:** prepare a spit poultice.
- **For leukorrhea:** prepare an infusion and use as a vaginal rinse.
- **As a bruise and wound healer:** prepare as a poultice, wash, or herbal bath.
- **Throat gargle and mouthwash:** prepare as an infusion for strep throat, lymphatic swelling, and gum inflammations.
- **For swollen glands and mastitis, varicose veins, and hemorrhoids:** prepare a poultice.
- **For oily skin:** create an astringent infusion and apply topically.
- **For herpes simplex, cold sores, and herpes zoster:** prepare a topical application as a poultice, tincture, or skin wash.

Self-heal is another edible plant. Although the taste is slightly bitter, the young shoots, leaves, and flowers can find their way into soups, salads, and stews while the bitters work to support optimal digestive function.

### Candida Wash
1 part Self-heal herb
1 part Marigold flowers
1 part Chamomile flowers

Prepare a strong infusion. Strain. Dilute with cooler but warm water. Pour into a douche bulb and use as a vaginal wash to relieve minor infection, irritation, and itching of common yeast infections or as a throat gargle for thrush.

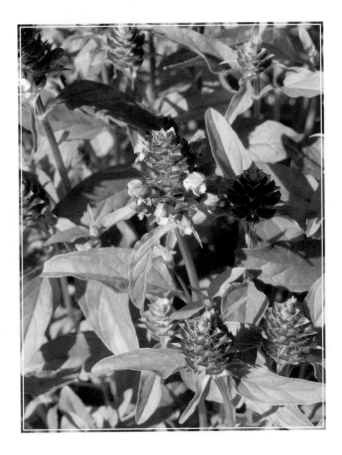

## Californian Poppy

The official state plant of California, Californian poppy can be found growing from Mexico through the United States and into northern BC, Canada. Its descriptive names, such as California sunlight and Cup of gold, remind us of the many varieties of human beings. Everyone is unique, with varieties of petals. Perhaps these bright petals welcome the sun with colors of orange, yellow, pink, or a deeper red, any of which quickly fold closed in the shade of the evening. People use the parts that grow above the ground for medicine, including the leaf, stem, and flowers.

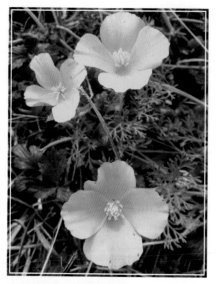

**Californian Poppy
(*Eschscholzia californica*)
Family: *Papaveraceae***

**Constituents:** alkaloids (such as eschscholtzine, sanguinarine, and protopine), flavonoids (rutin), carotenoids[179]

**Medicinal Action:** sedative, antispasmodic, antidepressant, antihistamine, analgesic, insomnia, bedwetting (incontinence), relaxing nervine, tension relief, antitussive

**Applications:** infusion, tincture

Consider a tea or tincture of California poppy for all variation of insomnia, of benefit for bedwetting in children to symptoms of hyperactivity and anxiety. California poppy can help calm the mind, uplift the spirits, promote relaxation, and alleviate worries in cases of mental exhaustion.

Its analgesic properties assist with pain management and its antispasmodic effects with nerve pain and toothaches, including the pain of shingles and sore muscles related to overexertion or arthritis.

**As a topical application for head lice:** when using the powdered dried leaves, mix with a little apple cider vinegar and apply as a paste to the scalp. Rinse out in the morning.

**A topical wash or poultice** made from the root is used for suppressing lactation after weaning a child from breast-feeding.

Although Californian poppy is a member of the poppy family and contains some sedative alkaloids, and distantly related to the famous opium poppy, this gentle plant contains no opium—it is a safe and effective nervine—if one is taking antidepressant medication then consult a health care professional. Avoid its use during pregnancy and breastfeeding.

### Antispasmodic Bronchitis Tea
1 teaspoon California Poppy herb
2 teaspoons Self-heal herb
2 teaspoons Daisy flower
1 teaspoon Sage leaf
½ teaspoon Caraway seed

Prepare as an infusion using 1 heaping teaspoon of mixture per cup of boiling water.

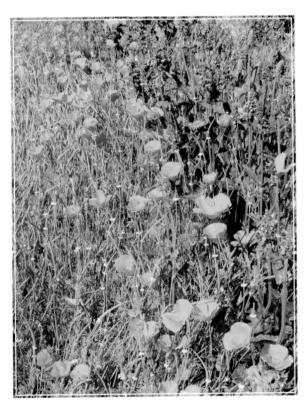

## Sage

When I see sage, I am immediately reminded of desert—dry weather and sagebrush, cowboy country. Sage is a tough plant that likes to grow in dry, arid, almost desert-like conditions and many species grow freely in the interior of British Columbia. Its astringent nature is drying, like its preference for dry soil and direct sun; it is drought-tolerant and hardy. The botanical name *Salvia* comes from the Latin word *salvere* meaning to be saved, or to be healed, which subtly speaks to the energetic powers of sage. Not so long ago, sage was listed in early twentieth-century drug pharmacopoeias for its medicinal value as a recognized medicine.

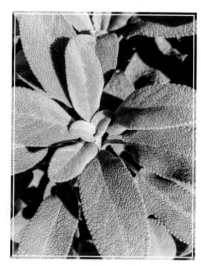

**Sage (*Salvia officinalis*)
Family: *Lamiaceae***

Try nibbling on the leaves of this Mediterranean native herb and discover the astringency, an immediate, tart, drying effect on the tongue. Crush the sage between your fingers and inhale the sharp fresh scent of volatile oils, used to sharpen the senses and take in the strongly pungent, smoky scent. It's quite intoxicating—medicine for the physical body as well as sacred spirit medicine.

There are numerous varieties of sage, generally used interchangeably, although the red sage, white, and green broad-leafed sage leaves are noted for highest medicinal value. Look for veins on both side of the leaf, with generally fuzzy, silvery, grey-green leaves set in pairs on the stalk. Sage blooms in the fall with purple-lipped petals wrapping around a fixed circular point on the stem. The aerial plant parts of leaf and stem are used medicinally.

**Chemical Constituents:** volatile oils (thujone, camphor), flavonoids (apigenin, diosmetin, and luteolin), bitters, flavonoids, and phenolic acids (ursolic, ellagic, rosmarinic acid, caffeic acids), tannins (salviatannin).[180,181]

The volatile oils are antioxidant and offer antibacterial properties as well. Historically, sage leaves were added into foods and meat to prevent spoilage, working as a natural preservative. The phenolic acids have been studied in vitro and have been found to be potent against Staphylococcus aureus, Escherichia coli, and Candida albicans. Rosmarinic acid is a potent antioxidant (due to the free radical scavenging catechols and caffeic acid).[182] The presence of phenolic acids is thought to contribute to the anti-inflammatory response by altering the concentrations of inflammatory messaging molecules.

**Medicinal Actions:** astringent, anti-inflammatory, antiseptic, antispasmodic, antiviral, emmenagogue, carminative, antioxidant, vermifuge, digestive, astringent

**Applications:** spice, infusion, tincture, honey, vinegar, syrup, wash, spray, body care, essential, ritual (smoke)

As a cognitive enhancer, research is looking into the nerve-protective benefits of sage for depression (possibly working through cholinesterase-inhibiting properties at least in vitro[183]), to enhance memory (in rats),[184] and in Alzheimer's disease.[185] Preliminary research and in vitro studies are confirming what traditional medicine has known and practiced for centuries by delving into the chemical workings of the plant to identify how its antioxidant properties work to reduce lipid peroxidation and offer neuroprotective properties. The volatile oils (particularly rosmarinic acid) in this plant are also part of its effectiveness.

Sage is a valuable women's herb for women transitioning through menopause and managing those unpredictable power surges that rush in by surprise and can distract from the focus at hand. Power surges have their positive side as well: they can be viewed as an opportunity to harness creative building energy within and direct it into a task at hand. This excess energy can be focused to spur change, the sharpened clarity of mind directed to social injustice or to influence policy changes; it's an opportunity for focused intention for a greater good.

Brew sage leaves as an infusion and cool. Steep ten minutes and then chill. Drink this tart blend cold for its abilities to reduce the intensity of those power surges and nighttime heat moments. Take in the opportunity to cultivate intention while sipping this refreshing bitter brew. A clinical trial conducted shows a significant 64 percent reduction in the number of hot flashes per day at the end of the two-month study.[186]

On many levels, sage is used for cleansing. It has a long history of ritual use for purifying one's physical space—both for the physical body and emotional field, for groups of individuals and for purifying one's environment. It is used with mindful intention prior to a sacred ceremony before initiating prayer and intention, to cleanse, remove negativity, and shift heavy, blocked energies to promote spiritual purification. Smudging with sage creates space for more positive possibilities in all realms and is used to align in harmony with the earth and with one's higher self. The smoke from sage is purifying and cleansing and is used to wash over that which can benefit from purification. While less frequently used, the smoke of plants has been applied throughout history for lung, nervous system, and skin issues, and to purify the air.[187] On our website, www.alchemyelixir.com, the white sage smudging wands are very popular, as well as the wands prepared from juniper boughs, sweetgrass, and cedar.

- **For bleeding of wounds, ulcers, and sores:** prepare a wash, poultice, or tincture.
- **For symptoms of hoarseness and a sore throat:** prepare infusion as a gargle or fresh sage juice.
- **For sprains and swellings:** a topical liniment or infusion can be applied directly to sprains and swellings.
- **For gum bleeding, inflammation, and dental abscess:** use a mouth rinse from an infusion or tincture.
- **For excessive bleeding (wounds or menstrual):** ingest tea or tincture and apply topical for external bleeding.
- **For asthma:** prepare a steam inhalation.
- **For the antiviral properties:** use a tincture, infusion, poultice, or diluted essential oil topically for cold sores.
- **For anti-lactation, to dry up milk after nursing:** prepare a topical poultice.
- **For bloating and indigestion:** prepare a carminative tea or ingest the tincture.
- **For intestinal infections:** the tincture is antiseptic and of benefit.
- **For head lice:** prepare a strong infusion with apple cider vinegar and apply as a hair rinse.
- **As a deodorant:** prepare an infusion in spray bottle with a couple drops of essential oils (Lavender or Rose Geranium Essential Oil).
- **For sinus congestion:** prepare a steam inhalation using the infused herb or drops of essential oil in a basin of hot water.
- **For symptoms of excessive sweating:** use an infusion applied topically in deodorant and ingested internally.

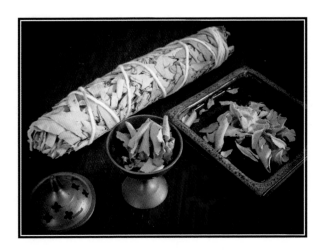

### Smudging

Light dried sage leaves or a sage bundle in a bowl or large shell (to collect the ashes), blow out the flame then use the smoke to smudge. Beginning in the northern corner, circulate the smoke into all four corners of a room and stagnant areas; smudge under chairs and furniture. Hold the intention of purification.

To smudge oneself or another, hold the highest intention of clearing away all that no longer serves one's higher self. Begin by washing your hands in the smoke, then direct the smoke around the heart (for heart purification), your mouth (to remind one of the importance of speaking respectfully), and around your hair (which protects your spirit). Then use the smoke to smudge from the head down to one's feet, smudging under the feet and then turning around and smudging the back of the body.

To smudge an object, lay it out on a table or a flat surface. Start at one end and gently fan the smoke across it, so that the smoke covers and flows across the entire piece. When it's done, let it sit for twenty-four hours.

Let the medicine continue to do its work; it will stop burning naturally (rather than dousing it with water). Remember to keep the burning embers contained safely until the wand stops burning.

The volatile oils in the herb contribute to its carminative nature, reducing gas, cramping, and indigestion, while the bitter components of the plant stimulate digestive function, encouraging intestinal mobility, the flow of bile, and pancreatic function.

**Cautions:** Avoid ingestion of sage during pregnancy and lactation (although it can be used at the time of weaning from breast-feeding to decrease milk production). Sage essential oil should not be taken internally.

### Power Surge Tea
2 teaspoons Sage leaf

Prepare as an infusion. Cool and drink 3–4 cups of tea per day.

### Raspberry Lavender Sage Lemonade
2 heaping teaspoons of Sage leaves
½–²/₃ cup Raspberries, fresh and muddled
1 tablespoon Lavender flowers
3 cups Water
Squeeze of fresh Lime juice (1 tablespoon)
Season with Honey (fennel or cinnamon honey is delicious) or Stevia leaves to taste

Boil the water and infuse the sage and lavender for 15 minutes. Strain. Mix in 1 teaspoon of honey and cool. Add in the muddled raspberries and lime and let sit covered overnight. Adjust the sweetness according to your taste buds and consume as a refreshing cold drink.

## Burdock Root

I look for the round, lavender, pur-plish, hooked flowers at the top of the plant and, as the name implies, burrs (hooked brackets in round colorful burrs that attach to clothing). Check out the hooks in the photo. Burdock (also called Gobo) can grow quite tall—three feet wide and eight to ten feet in height. The leaves are heart-shaped and waxy with cottony soft down on the underside. The long taproot is used

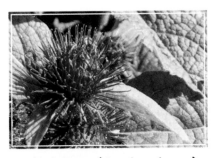

**Burdock Root (*Arctium lappa*)**
**Family: *Asteraceae***

medicinally in western herbal medicine and is harvested at the end of the first year of growth. Larger leaves may indicate a larger root. It is commonly found growing on park edges and sides of fields. The long taproot can be difficult to remove; hence its lack of popularity with gardeners. However, it is a welcome medicine to herb lovers.

**Constituents:** fatty acids, organic acids, phenolic acids, lignans, ses-quiterpenes, tannins, mucilage, inulin,[188] flavonoids, phytosterols, pectin, butyric and acetic acid[189]

**Medicinal Actions:** mineral-rich food, alterative, diaphoretic, blood puri-fier, gentle bitter and laxative, expectorant, diuretic, choleretic, antiseptic, blood sugar regulation

**Applications:** food, decoction, tincture, poultice, wash, fomentation, capsule

A popular root vegetable in other cultures, head into Chinatown to see this nutritious vegetable (Gobo resembles a parsnip). Once washed and peeled it can be added into stews, soups, and stir-fries (it absorbs the flavors around it). I frequently chop and add it into the pot of water with whole grains while cooking. When the grains are cooked so is the root, which can be ingested along with the grain. Pick the heart-shaped, large leaves and steam them like spinach.

As a nutritive tonic, 100 g of burdock root, cooked, offers 1.8 grams of Fiber, 49 mg of Calcium, 39 mg Magnesium, 360 mg Potassium, 0.9 ug Selenium, 2.6 mg Vitamin C, trace amounts of B Vitamins (niacin, thiamine, riboflavin, pantothenic acid, and pyridoxine), 20 ug Folate, and 14 mg Choline.[190]

Burdock is one of the most effective cleaners for the entire body; it supports the organs of elimination to remove toxicity in a number of ways. It is a diuretic herb, encouraging the elimination of uric acid and waste material from the kidneys, and a gentle yet effective laxative to enhance bowel function. It supports liver function, encourages elimination of toxins through the skin by encouraging sweating, and supports lymphatic function, effectively removing toxins through a variety of routes. Its slightly bitter properties promote digestion, including the release of hydrochloric acid from the stomach. Traditionally, burdock is known as an alterative herb, or blood cleanser, moving toxins from cellular storage into the bloodstream and encouraging elimination of waste matter from cells and organ systems. Reach for this herb for acne treatment and chronic skin eruptions including sores and itching dermatitis, for any condition of toxicity.

Through supporting kidney function, burdock will encourage removal of excess fluid and uric acid; it can be combined with anti-lithic herbs to assist with stone removal. It can also be used with analgesics and pain relievers for arthritis and gout.

Get to know this herb slowly—take your time—no one wants the symptoms associated with a quick, drastic approach to cleansing. If you choose to add it into your diet, start with a third of the daily adult dose and work up to the full amount over one to two weeks. It is an effective cleanser, so ingesting it slowly but steadily is the best approach. Ensure that your bowels are functioning daily to minimize the detox effects.

For arthritic joints, gout, and for individuals burdened with internal toxicity, add in regular consumption of vegetables, targeting the cruciferous vegetables, carrots, onion, watercress, chickweed, and nettles to supply trace nutrients to nourish the body, support detoxification, and ensure that the bowel and organs of elimination are working. Add in daily use of hot Epsom salt baths (see page 257) and dry skin brushing (page 240) to encourage lymphatic drainage and elimination.

I am all about an inviting spicy taste for bitter blends—they are friends for liver health, helping reduce a heavy toxin load on the liver, and are used for skin impurities and inflammation alike. This delicious warming blend is an ideal cleanser.

## Burdock's Bitter Blend – Skin Clear Tea

3 teaspoons Burdock root
3 teaspoons Dandelion root
1 teaspoon Cinnamon bark
1 teaspoon Licorice root
1 teaspoon Ginger root
1 teaspoon Fennel seed
½ teaspoon Stevia herb

Prepare as a decoction. Simmer covered on the stove for 15 minutes. Strain and drink 3 cups per day. If too sweet, decrease the amount of stevia.

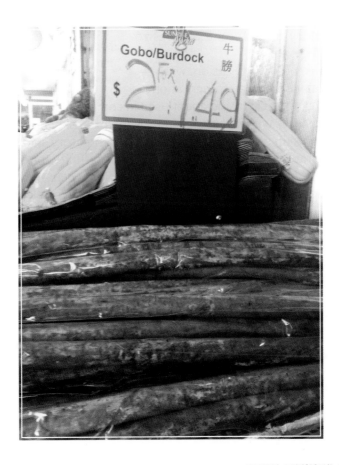

## Red Clover Herb

Red clover is a legume, actually, also known as clover flower, trefoil, and wild clover. The dried flower heads and leaves are used medicinally. It is often sowed in crop rotation for soil improvement and has been a long-known herbal medicine.

**Chemical Constituents:** isoflavones (formononetin,[191] genistan, daidzein and others), vitamins and minerals, flavonoids, volatile oils, coumarin, resin,[192] glucuronic acid, saponins, salicylic acids, fats, vitamins and minerals[193]

**Medicinal Actions:** antispasmodic, anti-inflammatory, expectorant, phytoestrogenic, alterative

**Applications:** poultice, infusion, wash, compress, poultice, vinegar, fomentation

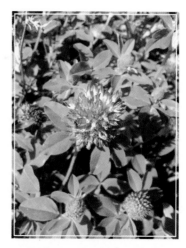

Red Clover Herb (*Trifolium pratense*) Family: *Leguminosae*

An effective blood cleansing agent used in combination with other alterative herbs in tea or tincture for improvement of skin disease, including irritated, scaling skin of psoriasis, sores, and inflammatory skin conditions, as well as respiratory conditions. With a particular affinity for childhood presentations of both eczema and asthma, red clover can assist two organ systems at once. Although it is not the main use today, red clover is an efficient expectorant and lung tonic herb for phlegm and congestion, difficulty breathing, allergies, and bronchitis. It also has a long history of use for cancer, congestion, tumors, cysts, and fibrous growths.

## Soothe My Cough Red Clover Expectorant

2 teaspoons Red Clover leaf and flower
1 teaspoon Plantain leaf
2 teaspoons Mullein leaf and flower
2 teaspoons Sweet Violet leaf

Use this as an expectorant herbal aid for decreasing spasms of a cough or bronchitis. For more flavor, add in 1 teaspoon of fennel.

Known as a phytoestrogen plant, red clover is not estrogenic. However, some of its chemical components are structurally similar to our bodies' own circulating estrogens. Phytoestrogens have the ability to fit into estrogen receptors and create a balancing effect, either reducing elevated estrogen levels or gently and weakly encouraging hormonal balancing in a deficient state. Red clover can be combined with hormone-balancing herbs for symptoms of menopause and premenstrual tension. Combine with yarrow and sage for those disruptive power surges at night.

**Topical applications:** prepare as a skin wash, external dressing, or poultice for wound care.

Consult an herbalist prior to use if taking blood thinners or statin medication due to potential blood thinning properties.

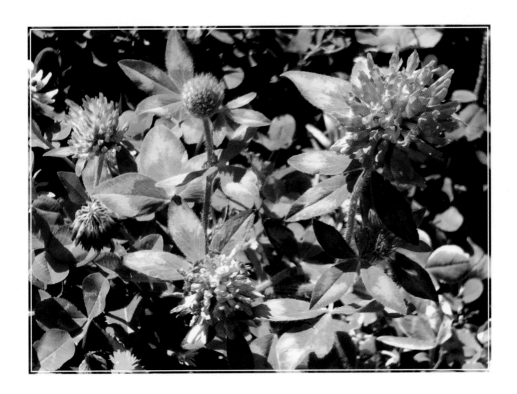

## Sweet Violet and Heartsease

Pansies and sweet violets are considered cousins, both belonging to the same genus, Viola. With the blooms lasting through spring until frost in cold, northern climates and through the entire winter in warmer regions, their cheery faces add brightness and joy to any garden. Their hundreds of species are often used interchangeably, with slight exception. Sweet violet, also known as blue violet or *Viola odorata*, is a native flower from Europe and said to be the original violet. It is primarily an expectorant for coughs and bronchial congestion. *Viola tricolor*, or pansies, is also known as miniature pansies, Johnny jumpers or jump ups (due to their ability to reseed themselves quite readily), and heartsease (due to the reputation of strengthening blood vessels). The dried flowers, leaves, and whole plant fresh are used medicinally.

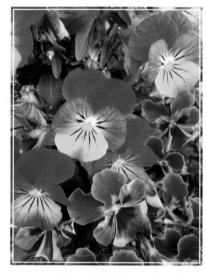

Sweet Violet (*Viola odorata*) and Pansies, Heartsease (*Viola tricolor*) Family: *Violaceae*

### How to distinguish between Violets and Pansies

According to the Horticultural Trades Association "the names 'pansy' and 'viola' are interchangeable for many . . . The way to tell the difference is that pansies have four petals pointing upwards and only one pointing down, while violas have three petals pointing up and two pointing down."[194] Others in the know just speak about the flower face and keep it simple. If the flower face or blooms are larger than five centimeters it is a pansy. If the flower face is smaller than five centimeters it is considered a violet. Pansies are derived from wild flowers and cultivated violas (considered the parent family).

## Comparison Chart: Pansies and Violets

### Pansies (Heartsease)
Tougher in winter, with a larger flower face, more rounded in shape; traditionally have more color variety (orange, blue, violet, white). Both species have blooms that can resemble a face, however the pansy has more contrast between the dark blotch (resembling a face) and main bloom color, and has more distinct markings.

### Violets
Violets or Blue violets have more flower blooms covering the entire plant and may be slightly smaller in size. That said, both plants can grow to the same size: three to four inches and five to six inches in the summer, so check out the blooms.

**Pansy or Heartsease: *Viola tricolor***

**Constituents:** flavonoids (quercetin, rutin, luteolin), saponin, gum, mucilage, bitter principles, phenolic acids (caffeic, salicylic acid)[195,196] tannins, coumarins[197]

**Medicinal Actions:** skin and mucous membranes, diuretic, anti-inflammatory, expectorant, alterative, antiallergic, antiacne, analgesic

**Applications:** infusion, tincture, poultice, wash, syrup, honey

**Viola tricolor:** considered more specific as an alterative and blood cleanser, spring tonic with slight laxative properties, used for skin conditions with oozing discharge (such as moist eczema), combines well with red clover. Think of this herb for children who suffer from both eczema and asthma, as the anti-inflammatory properties are also of benefit for the respiratory tract.

**Leaves:** A topical antimicrobial for skin problems such as boils, abscesses, skin ulcers, diaper rashes, insect bites, yeast, bruises, and rheumatism. Mash up the leaves and apply as a poultice or spit poultice. Known to be strengthening to the capillaries for varicose veins in a poultice, oil, or salve.

The presence of salicylic acid imparts pain-relieving properties. Prepare as a tea or use internally as a tincture for symptoms of dizziness and headaches.

## Heartsease Headache Relief Tincture
1 teaspoon dried Rosemary leaf
1 teaspoon dried Lavender flowers
1 teaspoon dried Heartsease herb and flowers

Prepare as a tincture (page 225) for pain and headache relief.

## Eczema Asthma Blend
2 parts Heartsease herb
2 parts Daisy flower
2 parts Chickweed herb
1 part Dandelion root
2 parts Cleavers herb
2 parts Red Clover leaf and flower

Prepare as an infusion using 1 heaping teaspoon of tea mixture to 1 cup of boiling water. Drink 2 to 4 cups daily.

This soothing alterative and anti-inflammatory blend offers support for the itching and heat of eczema, with special application for those with asthma and breathing difficulties as well as moist, weeping eczema.

### Sweet Violet: *Viola odorata*
Aerial plant part constituents: saponins, mucilage, flavonoids, phenolic glycosides,[198] volatile oil. Sweet violet is of use primarily for the lungs. The root, flowers, and leaves are used medicinally.

**Medicinal action:** circulatory and immune system stimulant, lymphatic, anti-inflammatory, mild antiseptic, antineoplastic and mild analgesic, soothing expectorant, urethritis and fibroids

**Applications:** infusion, tincture, poultice, wash, syrup, honey

The leaves are known for their antiseptic properties. Use as an alterative and mucous membrane tonic, anti-tussive, and for internal inflammations.

The root of the sweet violet offers strong expectorant and anti-inflammatory effects to loosen and remove phlegm from the lungs. Use for bronchitis, spastic coughing, and lung infections; gargle with the infusion for sore throat and mouth infections.

Preliminary research suggests that violas may help control the growth of certain cancers, such as breast and lung cancers,[199] possibly through antioxidant properties reducing the effects of oxidative stress.[200]

Both species are edible. Add in the flowers as a garnish to brighten any salad, into a smoothie or Perrier, or make Lavender mint lemonade and add in violet flowers for visual enhancement. Crystallized violets can make beautiful flower candies. Add to vinegar to impart color and fragrance, make into jam, or ferment to make sweet violet wine and delicious liquors. Sweet violets have also been used as a coloring agent for lotions and as a natural fabric dye, releasing a blue color upon infusion.

**Cautions:** When consumed in excessive amounts, the roots and seeds of sweet violet may cause nausea and vomiting. Start out with small doses.

## <u>Syrup of Fennel and Sweet Violet</u>

250 grams Violet flowers, dried
2 teaspoons Fennel seed
5 cups Water
Sugar

Pour 5 cups of boiling water over 250 grams dried violet flowers and leaves, add 2 teaspoons of fennel seeds and steep overnight. In the morning, strain, pour into a pot, and cook down to about half the liquid, stirring frequently to prevent boiling or burning. Reduce the liquid into a thick, syrup consistency. Measure and add equal the volume of sugar. Bottle and take off the spoon for symptoms of colds, bronchitis, and all breathing difficulties, or mix it into a tea blend.

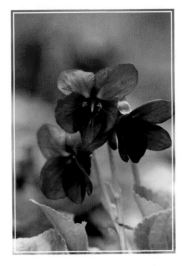

**Sweet Violet
(*Viola odorata*)**

## Cleavers Herb

Many common descriptive names for cleavers herb are due to its appearance. For example, it's named Clivers due to the many small hooks found on the entire herb. Also known as Goosegrass, a common food for geese and bed-straw (historically used as stuffing in mattresses) and actually thought to be one of the herbs used in the manger at Bethlehem.[201] Harvesting enthusiasts can recognize it by six

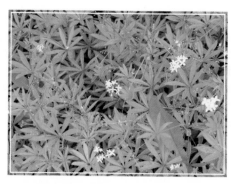

**Cleavers Herb (*Galium aparine*)**
**Family: *Rubiaceae***

to eight narrow leaves from one point, wrapping around the stem. Look for the rough hooks on the fragile, slender stalk. Gather the herb prior to it flowering, just before summer in late May, early June. The whole herb is used medicinally.

**Constituents:** anthraquinone, flavonoids (quercetin, rutin), iridoids, tannins, phenolic acids (salicylic, citric, caffeic acid derivatives), coumarins.[202] Cleavers contains caffeic acid and tannins, which contributes to the astringent effect that is useful as a gargle for sore throat related to a cold and also for diarrhea.

**Medicinal Actions:** blood cleanser and lymphatic, diuretic, for abnormal growth of tissue, anti-inflammatory, astringent, adaptogen tonic

**Applications:** infusion, tincture, poultice, fomentation, herbal vinegar, hair rinse

**Kidney Tonic and Diuretic:** Cleavers is useful as an effective diuretic for kidney and bladder complaints, for kidney stones, inflammation of the bladder (cystitis), and mild but recurrent urinary tract infections.

A lymphatic stimulant for enlarged lymph nodes and swollen glands, cleavers has traditionally been used for cancer for its ability to drain waste material from the kidneys. Cleavers is a versatile alterative and anti-inflammatory herb used internally for skin irritation including dermatitis, blemishes, psoriasis, and eruptions as well as a cleanser for arthritis. Incorporate the use of cleavers as a tea or tincture during seasonal cleansing and use external application (a poultice or fomentation) to provide relief to itchy skin inflammations, hard swellings, mumps, enlarged glands, bee stings, and burns. Traditionally a poultice of cleavers mixed with ground flaxseed or oatmeal powder was used topically over tumors. Use for anti-inflammatory support for bruising, sprains, and for healing abscesses, pustules, and boils. Cleavers historically has been prepared as an infusion and used as cleanser for the skin to lighten blotches, beauty spots, and freckles.

Some species of Cleavers (and older leaves) are very furry and irritating; other species with delicate tips are edible when the fresh leaf growth is cooked (sautéed or steamed).

## Lymphatic Tea
2 parts Cleavers herb
2 parts Red Clover leaf and flower
1 part Mullein leaf and flower
2 parts Sweet Violet herb and flowers

Prepare as an infusion. Drink for seasonal cleansing and detoxification for lymphatic congestion, mumps, swellings, and growths.

## Urinary Tract Infection Tea
1 part Corn Silk stigma
1 part Marigold herb
1 part Plantain herb
1 part Cleavers herb

Prepare as an infusion using 1–2 teaspoons of tea mixture per cup of boiling water.

## Teen Acne Support
2 teaspoons Nettle leaf
1 teaspoon Burdock root
1 teaspoon Cleavers herb
1 teaspoon Dandelion leaf
2 teaspoons Red Clover leaf and flower
½ part Spearmint herb
½ part Stevia herb

Prepare as an infusion using 1 teaspoon of tea mixture per cup of boiling water.

## Rosemary Herb

The common names of this plant are simply majestic and inviting: rosemary has been called rosemarie and rosmarine, and its Latin root *ros marinus* translates to "dew of the sea." Although the leaves are slightly leathery, both the leaf and blue-purple flowers can be used for flavoring in food, while the leaves and thin twigs are used as medicine. The stalk is not used, being rather woody.

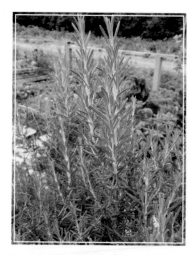

**Constituents:** volatile oil (camphor, limonene, linalool and others), flavonoids (apigenin, luteolin), rosmarinic acids, and phenolic acids,[203] terpenoids[204]

**Rosemary Herb (*Rosmarinus officinalis*) Family: *Lamiaceae***

**Medicinal Actions:** nervine tonic, antiseptic, antifungal, antimicrobial, diaphoretic, analgesic, antispasmodic, anti-inflammatory, antioxidant, carminative, liver tonic, astringent, circulatory support

**Applications:** infused oil, infusion, poultice, gargle, tincture, honey, vinegar, essential oil, wash, fomentation, liniment, hair rinse, body care, infused oil

Rosemary is a supportive herb for many body systems. It can be considered a nervous system tonic for low energy, menopause, and stress-related conditions.[205] I consider it a pick-me-up tonic to uplift the spirits, for mild depression and to assist the body in dealing with long-term stress. Rosemary and lavender create ideal support during times of transition, supporting the body's ability to gracefully adapt to change. For cognitive function, to assist with memory recall, and improve circulation in the body (encouraging blood flow to all areas and its flavonoids and antioxidants can assist with keeping capillaries strong), reach for rosemary. Most people are familiar with the characteristic scent of Rosemary due to its volatile oils. Simply crushing the leaf and inhaling the scent can offer a rapid increase in alertness. It is a useful essential oil to have on hand when studying, as it enhances mental clarity.

Rosemary can be used as an antioxidant herb, while the antiseptic and anti-inflammatory effects of its volatile oils make it an ideal application for open wounds and for infection. A mild pain reliever, it offers relief for leg cramps, persistent tight muscles, sore muscles, headaches, and nerve-related issues such as sciatica. The flavonoids of rosemary offer support for fragile capillaries, for varicose veins, and hemorrhoids.

The volatile oils in the leaf work as a digestive for symptoms of indigestion as well as to support liver function. Being slightly astringent, rosemary can be of benefit prepared in a tea infusion for a throat gargle, or drink to calm down diarrhea and offer protection against food poisoning.

Rosemary is antiviral and can be used for a cold or flu, or for other viral conditions such as epstein barr, mononucleosis, cold sores, and influenza. It encourages improved circulation, also ideal for a cold and for warming cold hands and feet. Its antifungal properties provide use as a foot soak for athlete's foot, a mouth rinse for oral thrush, or for a yeast infection.

Rosemary can be used as a spice and food seasoning. Try mixing it into potatoes, mushroom and meat dishes, or add it into herbal honeys or vinegars. The antioxidant properties, namely rosmarinic acid and carnosic acid, prevent oxidation of fats and oil; thus rosemary can extend the shelf life of a product, working as a natural preservative without the toxic and carcinogenic effects of many laboratory preservatives like BHT and BHA (butylated hydroxytoluene, butylated hydroxyanisole).[206]

**Cautions:** Although rosemary has a long history of use in body care and cosmetic use, there are rare occurrences of contact dermatitis from extended contact with the fresh leaves. Outside of normal food ingestion, avoid large amounts during pregnancy, especially the first trimester and avoid the use of rosemary essential oil in circumstances of seizures or epilepsy. This is a potent plant, so excessive ingestion is unnecessary.

- **As a hair rinse:** form a strong infusion and apply to the scalp to stimulate circulation, improve hair growth, and prevent dandruff.
- **For gum inflammation, canker sores, and bad breath:** prepare a mouthwash from an infusion or diluted tincture.
- **For oily or acne-prone skin:** prepare an infusion and use as an astringent face rinse.
- **For a sore throat and tonsillitis:** prepare an infusion and use as a throat gargle.
- **For nail fungus and athlete's foot:** prepare an infusion and use as a foot soak and antifungal agent.
- **As a herbal bath:** use as an invigorating pick-me-up stimulant.
- **For healing of cuts and open wounds:** Apply an infusion as a skin wash.
- **For sinus congestion:** prepare an herbal steam.
- **For headache support:** prepare an infusion or tincture.

## Rosemary Oregano Head Lice Blend

1 teaspoon dried Rosemary leaves
1 teaspoon Oregano herb
150 ml Apple Cider Vinegar
10 drops Tea Tree Essential Oil

Infuse herbs in apple cider vinegar for 4 days. Strain and add in essential oil. Use as a hair rinse, keeping on the hair overnight. Use a lice comb to work through hair. Have the child sleep on a towel and then shampoo out in the morning.

## Thyme Herb and Leaf

The name thyme is derived from the Latin name *thymus*, traced back to the Greek name *thymos,* meaning spirited. Thyme is a much-respected herb associated with bravery and strength, historically gifted to soldiers heading to battle. Dried thyme bundles can be burned for imparting a sense of courage while unleashing the strong, smoky, antiseptic nature of thyme. Historically, thyme was added into foods as a seasoning spice, an ingredient in liqueurs, and was used to both prevent and assist in overthrowing food poisoning. It has a long history of use during the times of the plague to ward off illness. Harvest leaves in the morning, before the plant flowers in the summer.

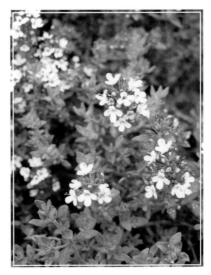

**Thyme Herb and Leaf (*Thymus vulgaris*) Family: *Lamiaceae***

**Constituents:** volatile oils (thymol, carvacrol), tannins, flavonoids,[207] triterpenoid saponins, resins

**Medicinal Actions:** antiseptic, antibacterial, antiviral, antioxidant, antifungal, expectorant, anticandida, vermifuge, carminative, anti-tussive, antispasmodic, diaphoretic, rubefacient

**Applications:** infusion, infused oil, essential oil, tincture, fomentation, poultice, honey, syrup, steam

This infection-fighting plant is packed full of volatile oils, which contribute to its antiseptic properties: the thymol and carvacrol are disinfectant to the mucous membranes of the lungs and kidneys as they are excreted from the body. Thyme offers valuable antimicrobial support for gut infections, including food poisoning, and those unwanted yet common childhood parasites (such as pin worms and thread worms).

In addition to the antibacterial and antiviral properties, thyme is an expectorant herb: it loosens thick, sticky phlegm and creates a productive cough for removal of copious amounts of mucous. It is known especially for combatting a dry cough with raw mucous membranes, as it produces a protective covering over the dry membranes and assists the productivity of the cough. It is useful for asthma, bronchitis, and breathing issues. Consider this a useful antiviral and diaphoretic herb for a cold or flu. Create a syrup of rose hips, yarrow, and mint as a "flu therapy on a spoon" or use thyme in an herbal steam for congestion using the two teaspoons of herb of thyme and two to three drops of lemon essential oil in a basin of boiling water. Its antispasmodic properties make this an ideal home remedy for sporadic convulsive coughs, thickened mucous, and inflammation of the bronchial tubes in cases of bronchitis. It also provides benefit topically for aching joints and muscle spasms related to rheumatism and arthritis.

The highly astringent nature, due to the tannin content, makes thyme an option for diarrhea, especially related to foreign bacteria in the gut, and a topical antiseptic for cuts.

Thyme is both a bitter and carminative herb for supporting digestion: prepare an herbal vinegar, tea, or tincture for symptoms of diarrhea, gastritis, colic, and gas. Its bitter nature is used to stimulate digestion and support liver function.

- **For skin fungus, viral infections (warts and shingles), and antiseptic wound care:** prepare a disinfectant skin wash.
- **For tight muscles, athletic injuries and rheumatic issues such as arthritis and inflammation:** use a poultice, liniment, or topical applications.
- **For strep throat and candida infections of the mouth:** prepare an infusion and use as a gargle.
- **For ear infections:** prepare an infused oil and use for ear drops or poultice.
- **For sinus congestion, asthma, allergies, and colds:** prepare an infusion and use as a steam inhalation.
- **For leukorrhea or candida fungal infection:** prepare as an herbal wash.
- **For mastitis:** combine with plantain and prepare as a poultice.
- **For cold and flu symptoms, congestion, and body aches:** prepare an infusion as a steam or herbal bath.

Thyme is a strong tasting herb with a potent, sharp aroma—a warning for its potent nature. Due to its strong taste, it is rare to over ingest, however it is important to note that this herb was never intended to be used in excessive amounts and care is especially required during pregnancy. If using the essential oil topically, it should be well diluted or may cause skin irritation.

## Thyme and Juniper Muscle Ease Liniment

1 tablespoon dried Thyme herb
1 tablespoon dried Rosemary leaves
2 tablespoon dried Juniper berries, crushed
1 teaspoon dried Ginger root
200 ml Grape-seed Oil
½ cup unrefined Coconut Oil
4–6 drops Rosemary Essential Oil

Prepare an infused oil using the dried herbs of thyme, rosemary, ginger and juniper berries infused in the grape-seed oil. Heat on a low temperature following instructions on page 233. Strain. When just barely warm, mix in ½ cup coconut oil and rosemary essential oil. Pour into a salve container. Chill to harden. Apply as a topical rub for arthritis, swelling, and stiffness.

## Oregano

Oregano is a popular remedy on the market in the last couple of years and another example of Mother Nature's potent medicines. Perhaps most widely known for its antimicrobial properties, oregano can be used to address infections like H pylori infections, Candida, opportunistic parasite infections, fungus such as athlete's foot, and respiratory and skin infections. Oregano is native to the Mediterranean and is recognized

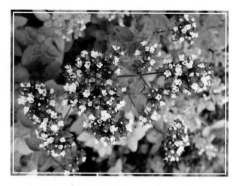

**Oregano (*Origanum vulgare*)**
**Family: *Lamiaceae***

by its white and pink flowers and tiny green leaves. The leaves and seeds are used medicinally.

Used frequently as an immune tonic for labored and difficult breathing and symptoms of a cold and flu, the potency of this herb is not in question; however, it is important to be clear of the modes of application. The tea and tincture of oregano is available for ingestion in small dosages. The essential oil of oregano is very strong and needs to be extremely diluted in a base oil prior to topical use. Oregano, in correct administration, provides antibacterial properties against gram positive and negative bacteria, including *Salmonella*, *Escherichia coli*, and *Staphylococcus*, and many other growing risks of antibiotic-resistant infections.[208] The chemical constituents carvacrol and thymol are most concentrated in the essential oil and are responsible for the antioxidant, antimicrobial, and antifungal actions. Oregano, prepared as an infusion or tincture, offers effective antiseptic support for urinary tract and lung infections as well as gum inflammation and indigestion. The volatile oils from a tea are carminative in nature, good for digestive upset and trapped abdominal gas.

**Constituents:** volatile oils containing phenols (carvacrol, thymol, pinene), phenolic acids (rosmarinic acids, caffeic acid), flavonoids, saponins, bitter principles[209]

**Medicinal Actions:** antifungal, antibacterial, antioxidant, antispasmodic, antimicrobial, antiseptic, carminative, analgesic

**Applications:** infusion, tincture, liniment, poultice, fomentation, infused oil, vinegar, honey, salve, essential oil

Prepare a strong infusion as an antiseptic for a sore throat and gargle several times throughout the day. Ingest the tea for symptoms of a cold and drink to relieve an elevated fever. Keep the tea covered until ready for use and inhale the potent volatile oils to open up the sinus passages.

Use as a topical preparation, as an antispasmodic and pain relief herb for general aches, muscle pains, rheumatism, and arthritis. Topically, the effect of oregano is rubefacient, sending fresh blood flow to localized tissues and working as an antiseptic wash for open wounds and sores.

**Caution:** May be irritating to the skin and mucous membranes for susceptible individuals—try on a small area with a reduced dose first. Avoid use during pregnancy.

## Decongestant Oregano Coconut Vapor Rub

1 drop Oregano Essential Oil
1 drop Lemon Essential Oil
1 tablespoon unrefined Coconut Oil

Mix with a spoon and bottle or mix into a liquid. The texture is best hardened for a topical rub. Test on a small area of skin first before using this as a chest rub for seasonal allergies and congestion. It can also be rubbed onto the nostrils to hydrate dry skin; the volatile oils will assist with clearing the sinus passages for easier breathing. When experiencing the initial symptoms of a cold, I suggest to clients to rub this mixture onto the soles of their feet prior to heading off to bed. The volatile oils will be absorbed through the thin skin on the arch of the foot and will disinfect the lungs, enhancing immune activity while sleeping; this simple application alone can go a long way in warding off a cold. Keep in mind that essential oils are highly concentrated and should be well diluted. If your skin is sensitive, increase the amount of coconut oil in the blend.

## Oregano Antiviral Throat Spray

½ teaspoon Oregano herb
½ teaspoon Sage leaf
½ teaspoon Self-heal herb
½ teaspoon Spearmint herb
1 teaspoon organic Lemon rind, grated

½ cup boiling Water
¼ cup Brandy
2–3 tablespoons Vegetable glycerine
3–5 drops Tea Tree Essential Oil

Prepare a strong infusion using ½ cup of boiling water to pour over the herbs. Steep covered for 15 minutes. Strain. Add in the ¼ cup of brandy, 2–3 tablespoons of vegetable glycerine, and 3–5 drops of tea tree essential oil. Mix together well. Pour into 2 two-ounce spritzer bottles. Spritz into the mouth frequently during the day to relieve symptoms of a sore throat. The lemon astringency and the antiviral herbs are a welcome soothing relief for viral infections as well as gum inflammation and dry mouth.

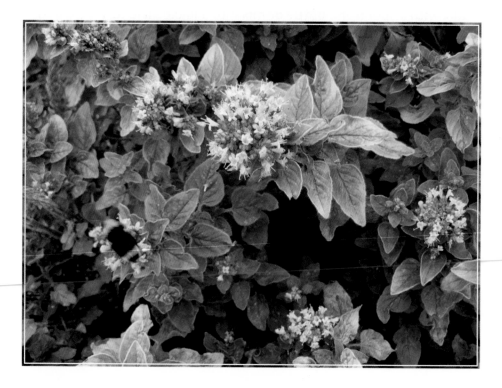

## Red Raspberry Leaf

Wild and garden-cultivated red raspberry bushes offer tasty berries packed full of flavonoids and beneficial immune-enhancing properties, while the leaves offer valuable medicine for the female reproductive system. In fact, it is such a women's herb that the leaves can be used as a tonic throughout the reproductive years, from the teenage years to the childbearing years and through menopause.

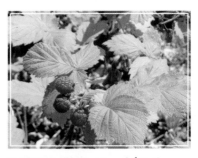

**Red Raspberry Leaf (*Rubus idaeus*) Family: *Rosaceae***

**Chemical Constituents of fruit:** citric and malic acid, flavonoids (including rutin), tannins,[210] volatile oil, pectin, ferric citrate, fragarine. According to herbalist Ruth Trickey in her book *Women, Hormones & The Menstrual Cycle*, these constituents are "responsible for uterine tonic effect . . . possessing contradictory effects—on one hand relaxing the uterine muscle and on another initiating contractions. This has confounded researchers, but confirmed herbalists' beliefs in raspberry leaves as a uterine tonic."[211]

**Chemical Constituents of leaf:** flavonoids and tannins and nutrients including vitamin C and A, iron, calcium, and selenium.[212]

In 100 g, the fruit or Raspberry contains: 6.5 g of dietary Fiber, 25 mg Calcium, 22 mg Magnesium, 151 mg Potassium, 29 mg Phosphorus, 26 mg Vitamin C, 33 IU Vitamin A, 136 ug Lutein, 12 ug Beta-carotene, 0.67 mg Manganese, 7.8 ug Vitamin K.[213]

Raspberry leaf tea provides a rich source of vitamins and minerals and can be drunk as a daily tonic for iron deficiency anemia combined with other iron-rich herbs like nettle and alfalfa.

**Medicinal Actions:** uterine tonic herb, astringent for a sore throat, mouthwash, bleeding, both a laxative and for diarrhea, nosebleeds, galactagogue, a fertility enhancer and female tonic during pregnancy (partus preperator), to prevent miscarriage, emmenagogue, prevent hemorrhage during birth

**Applications:** infusion, tincture, gargle, skin wash, syrup, poultice, eyewash

One of the chemical constituents, fragarine, has been found to strengthen uterine muscles and show effects that continue to perplex and mystify scientists, offering two contradictory effects in the body. During pregnancy, fragarine induces a regulating action, ensuring a relaxing effect on the pregnant uterus, and when the uterine muscle is relaxed the herb can induce contractions; hence fragarine both relaxes the uterus and promotes contractions. Perhaps as a balancer it simply knows how to work as needed in the moment.

Red raspberry leaf is perhaps one of the most renowned female reproductive tonics, with centuries of use for women's health, dating back to the early 1500s, it is used as a hormone regulator in the teenage years and a hormone balancer. However, it is most well-known for its tonic effects to prepare the body for a safe pregnancy. Red raspberry can be blended with chaste tree berry, yarrow, red clover, or motherwort for monthly hormonal support and mixed with lady's mantle to minimize excessive bleeding. It can also be combined with chaste tree and nettle for a teenage reproductive tonic. This is one of nature's balancers for reproductive well-being.

As a pregnancy tonic, red raspberry leaf tea offers outstanding support throughout the entire nine months of pregnancy, ** strengthening the uterine muscles for ease of childbirth and ensuring a smooth, healthy pregnancy and a safe delivery.

In line with its balancing nature, red raspberry can tone the uterine muscles for an easier childbirth. During labor, the herb can assist with regulating uterine contractions to more effectively speed up delivery; it does not increase contractions per se but simply supports what the body is already doing and thus may be used to shorten labor. The tannin-rich leaf can help reduce the risk of excessive bleeding and hemorrhage. After birth, consuming red raspberry tea can facilitate the uterus in returning to its former size and assist with balancing rapidly fluctuating hormones. Numerous animal studies show that manganese deficient females showed a lack of maternal instinct and outright indifference to their offspring. When supplemented with the mineral manganese, they again developed maternal interest in caring for their offspring. Raspberry leaves contain manganese which may help prevent this phenomenon and strengthen maternal instinct.

**The centuries of this plant's use assures its safety throughout pregnancy. There are rare circumstances involving extremely toned women with strong pelvic muscles where raspberry may be too stimulating in the first trimester. In this case, lower your dose or set this herb aside for the first trimester and resume in the last months of pregnancy. [214]

The fresh fruit have a weak laxative effect, as do other berries, such as blackberries and rosehips. Blackberries are from the same family, are highly astringent, and can be made into a strong syrup for digestive regularity; plant parts are also binding for loose bowel movements.

- **For menstrual cramps:** combine with ginger and ingest as an infusion or tincture.
- **As an eyewash:** prepare as an infusion with chamomile and marigold and carefully strain.
- **For allergies, sinus congestion, and copious mucous:** blend with goldenrod and nettles in tea or tincture form.
- **For antidiarrheal effects:** combine with cinnamon and plantain to reduce fluid and tone mucous membranes in a tea or tincture form.
- **To reduce symptoms of a sore throat:** use as an infusion for a throat gargle.
- **For inflammation of gingivitis, and bleeding gums after flossing:** prepare an infusion and use as a mouth rinse.
- **For candida and symptoms of leukorrhea:** prepare a strong infusion as a vaginal wash.
- **For skin lacerations, burns, raw, open sores and swollen veins:** combine with plantain and self heal. An external skin wash can be used.
- **For large pores and acne:** prepare an astringent face toner.
- **As a lactation stimulant:** mix with fennel seed and prepare as an infusion.

## Monthly Mineral Rich Hormone Tonic
1 teaspoon dried Red Raspberry leaf
1 teaspoon dried Nettle leaf
2 teaspoons dried Dandelion leaf
1 teaspoon dried Dandelion root

Use 1 teaspoon per cup of water. Prepare an infusion for daily use as a tea. Use for a couple months to assist with regulating menstrual cycles and to minimize fluid retention and liver congestion.

## Borage

The medicinal use of borage is documented as far back as 40–90 AD when Dioscorides, a botanist, doctor, and pharmacist, wrote about this vibrant, bright blue flower as a plant used to brighten the spirits. Use when feeling blue, especially when there is mental exhaustion and much physical stress involved. Borage grows wild and is also welcome in any garden. The bright blue flowers can be added into a salad or sprinkled into a fruit salad, while the leaves can also be eaten, tasting somewhat like cucumber.[215] The flowers and leaves are used medicinally.

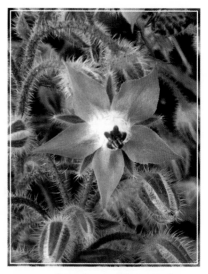

**Borage (*Borago officinalis*)**
**Family: *Boraginaceae***

**Constituents:** mucilage, fatty acids, saponins, tannins, pyrrolizidine alkaloids (in very small amounts,[216] "reported as 0.01% and 2 to 10 ppm for dried samples"[217])

**Medicinal Actions:** adrenal support adaptogen, mood enhancer, galactagogue, emollient, demulcent, diaphoretic, expectorant, anti-inflammatory, nervine

**Applications:** infusion, tincture, poultice, infused oil, body care, infused oil

For adrenal support, borage nourishes, promoting a calm body and mind, uplifting the spirits. Used for mild depression and hormonal-associated mood swings, it is a pick-me-up plant when one is feeling blue from elevated stress and subsequent exhaustion. An adaptogen tonic herb for adrenal overwork, borage assists the body in adapting to changes in one's internal and external world, helping with regulation of the parasympathetic and sympathetic nervous system. Consider borage during the transition of menopause or even for general anxiety. Traditionally borage was used for digestive complaints, but it can be used to minimize leaky gut syndrome, for inflammation of the stomach and intestines, and for conditions of colitis, irritable bowel, and ulcers.

An infusion of the leaf provides mucilage support for the lungs and kidneys, providing an expectorant effect in the lungs while removing excess mucous and soothing the urinary tract. Combine with herbs for the lungs and kidneys for a complete formulation.

The infused oil of borage offers rich nourishing support for dry, aging skin, itchy skin, eczema, and dermatitis. Consider creating this from the dried flowers or preparing a poultice with fresh or dried herbs to apply over rashes for a rich, topical massage oil for whole body application.

**Mindfulness:** Avoid excessive consumption of this cheery plant. The herb has a long history of documented use; however, consider it for short-term support at a low dosage and avoid use during pregnancy. Avoid administration to infants and choose other amazing plants for support if one has a pre-existing liver condition or is taking hepatotoxic medication.

## Borage Happiness Tea
2 tablespoons Borage flowers
1 tablespoon Rose petals
1 teaspoon Lavender flowers
1 tablespoon Lemon balm
½ teaspoon Spearmint

Prepare an infusion using 1 healing teaspoon of tea mixture to 1 cup of boiling water. Serve with fresh borage flowers in the tea for a pick-me-up, gentle mood elevator, and relaxing blend.

## Borage Irritable Bowel Blend

1 teaspoon Borage flowers
1 teaspoon Chamomile flowers
1 teaspoon Plantain leaves
1 teaspoon Hops strobiles
½ teaspoon Peppermint leaves

Prepare an infusion. Drink 3–4 cups daily for short-term assistance with cramping, gastric irritation, and spasms.

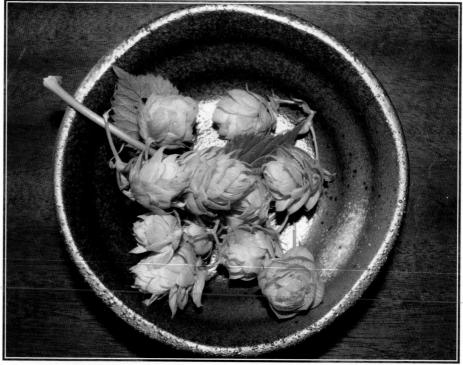

**Hops:** *Humulus lupulus*

## Hops

Hops have been used since ancient times for beer brewing. Today, we know that the bitter principles of humulon contribute to the characteristic bitter taste in the beverage and are added in for preservative, antimicrobial, and antibiotic properties.[218,219]

Hops are found interlaced around hedges and gates and are a welcome visual to any garden. The layered cone-shaped fruit, also known as the dried strobile of the female plant, is used medicinally. To recognize the yellow or light-green strobile, look for "layered" petals around a pinecone shape.

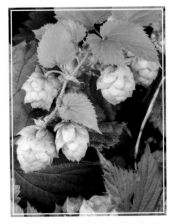

**Hops (*Humulus lupulus*)**
**Family: *Cannabaceae***

**Constituents:** volatile oils (humulene, myrcene), flavonoids, resins with bitter principles (valeronic acid, lupamaric acid (humulone) and lupulinic acid—when dried converting into the sedative isovaleric acid), tannins,[220] isoflavones (formononetin)[221]

**Medicinal Actions:** mild sedative, hypnotic, bitter digestive, analgesic

**Applications:** infusion, tincture, capsule, herbal bath, herbal sleep pillow

There is a bit of a debate, and a great deal of misunderstanding over the presence of estrogen-like compounds in hops. Some studies confirm[222] the presence of phytoestrogens, and other studies confirm their absence. Through historical observation of European hop-pickers, however, much was learned about the properties of the plant, leading to an understanding of the endocrine and hormonal properties; female hop-pickers experiencing hormonal changes due to the isoflavones contained within. The very weak phytoestrogenic properties of hops (isoflavones are also found in red clover, soy, fennel, tempeh, beans, and lentils) can be a welcome addition for support for early menopause, in circumstances of lack of ovulation, and for amenorrhea (absent menstruation).

The term phytoestrogen speaks to a chemical structure found in some plants, including red clover. It is similar enough to bind to the various estrogen receptors in our bodies, yet far weaker in strength and not completely identical to estrogen. Modern research is showing that phytoestrogens offer some balancing properties, mildly mimicking estrogen, resulting in a net increase in estrogen if and when needed. Yet it is also antiestrogenic, acting to lower overall estrogen levels (an antiestrogen effect),[223] When converted by the body into substances that weakly resemble estrogens, it competes for binding sites by filling estrogen receptors; thus phytoestrogens can result in the reduction in overall net exposure to estrogens. In her book *The Natural Menopause Handbook*, Amanda McQuade Crawford, MNIMH, writes that "Traditional herbal remedies that have helped alleviate female problems caused by high estrogen are known to contain phytoestrogens. Continuing research suggest that these herbs do not always increase a women's estrogen. Herbs with plant hormones do not behave like hormone drugs."[224] Science is investigating protective qualities of isoflavones against certain types of cancer, including that of the bowel and breast.[225] Plant phytoestrogen's potencies are estimated to be "approximately 1000-fold weaker than that of estradiol (the primary female sex hormone),"[226,227] further contributing to the lowered net estrogen effect.

Hops are mildly sedating and relaxing, used for tension, exhaustion, headache and restlessness. Use a combination of hops and Californian poppy for insomnia. Hops have been said to "shorten the time it takes to fall asleep and deepen the slumber."[228] Prepare a tincture for a more concentrated dose. In addition to its nervous system relaxant properties, hops are also antispasmodic for cramping of the digestive system; their slightly bitter notes gently stimulate and support optimal digestion and enhance liver detoxification functions.

Hops are also diuretic; this is thought to be due to the chemical constituent asparagine.

**Caution:** Those on antidepressant medications should avoid hops. Contact dermatitis has been reported due to the pollen and possibly the volatile oils.

### Hops California Poppy Nervine Tincture
Brandy or Vodka
Hops strobiles
California poppy herb and flower

Use equal portions and pack into a glass jar. Cover with brandy or vodka. Prepare as a tincture as on page 225. Strain and use after 2 weeks. Use for symptoms of anxiety, worries during the day, and sleeplessness at night. The adult dose varies between 2–4 ml, 2–5 times daily. Take at night for insomnia.

## Hops Bitter Blend

2 parts Hops strobiles
2 parts Dandelion root
1 part Marigold flower
½ part Caraway seed

Prepare as a tincture. Take 2.5–5 ml in a shot glass of warm water prior to meals for optimal digestion, stimulating gastric juices and releasing digestive enzymes.

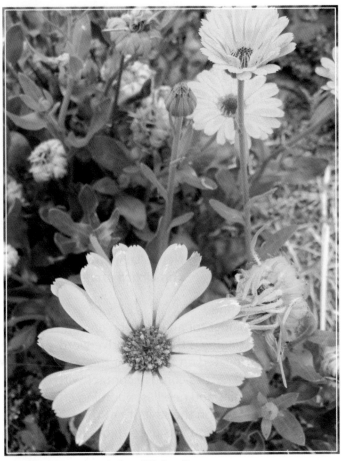

**Marigold: *Calendula officinalis***

# Plants to Gather

## Nettle Leaf and Herb

Nettles are one of my fondest herbal friends. Each spring, I look forward to steaming nettle leaves like spinach and flavoring them with coconut oil. Nettles are known by herbalists as *the* tonic herb for supporting the entire body and all organ systems. Rosemary Gladstar, one of the grandmothers of modern herbal medicine, often says "if you don't know what else to do, use nettles!" There is truth to this statement!

If you frequent open woodlands or have walked on the sides of a field, you likely will know about nettles. Stinging nettles are recognizable by the serrated edges of their leaves, tiny stinging hairs on the whole plant surface, and their height of one to three feet. A gentle reminder for anyone who encounters stinging nettle along a path or in a field: *stinging* is the descriptive word. Fresh nettles are not gentle. Tiny fine hairs located on the tips of the leaves sting, releasing formic acid, and when fresh nettles come in contact with the skin, there will be localized tingling and a pins and needles, numbing effect that can last minutes or hours depending upon the severity of the sting. It is not harmful, just uncomfortable. This action was used traditionally for symptoms of arthritis as a counterirritant to relieve pain-filled joints. The bite of these

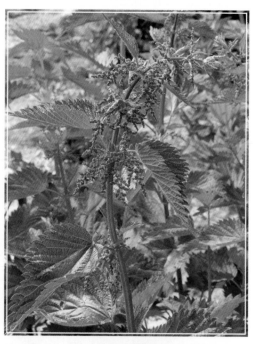

**Nettle Leaf and Herb (*Urtica dioica* and *Urtica urens*) Family: *Urticaceae***

hairs are deactivated when tinctured, cooked, steamed, frozen, juiced, or dried. Despite its name, this edible plant makes a delicious medicine either as a culinary food, dried for teas, or tinctured.

**To harvest in the spring:** Wear gloves, select tender young nettles about one to one-and-a-half feet tall and clip the fresh shoots and delicate stalk. Taller, mature plants are less palatable since the stem becomes too woody to eat, but the leaves are still valuable. The entire aerial plant parts, stem and leaves, are used medicinally. The roots also have their value for benign prostate enlargement by "inhibiting binding activity of sex hormone binding globulin."[229]

When wild crafting, leave a number of fresh shoots in every grove to ensure that the plants have an opportunity to reseed in the fall and you will have herbs to harvest for the future! Leave the first plants and the last plants in a grove—harvest only from the center. Sustainable wild crafting techniques are essential for ensuring a continuation of your wild harvest.

**Constituents:** chlorophyll, vitamin C, serotonin, histamine,[230] acids (formic acid, silicic acid, fumaric acid), flavonoids, tannin, lignans,[231] and packed full of minerals including carotenoids, calcium, iron, silica, and chlorophyll.[232] 100 g of blanched Nettle leaves provide 6.9 g dietary Fiber, 481 mg of Calcium, 1.64 mg Iron, 57 mg Magnesium, 334 mg Potassium, 14 ug Folate, 2011 IU Vitamin A, and 498 ug of Vitamin K.[233] Nettle leaf can be consumed as a nutritive, tonic food and for conditions of iron deficiency anemia. It can be consumed for extended periods of time by individuals who are depleted or recovering from a long illness.

**Medicinal Actions of leaf and stem:** alterative, whole body cleanser, nutritive mineral-rich tonic, antiallergic, diuretic, galactagogue, antihemorrhage, antirheumatic

**Medicinal Actions of root:** prostate enlargement

**Applications:** infusion, tincture, nutritive, food, herbal vinegar, hair rinse, syrup, juice, lotion

An alterative tonic herb, otherwise known as a blood cleanser, supports the elimination of waste material out of the body and supports liver and kidney function. Nettle leaf is *the* herb for all types of skin conditions: blemishes, rashes, hives, and itching. Consume as a fresh juice, tincture, or tea for dry, irritated eczema, psoriasis, and scaling skin eruptions. Drink daily as a tonic for adolescent acne or as a nourishing tonic for whole body health, packed full of nutrients while purifying the blood.

For allergy relief there is nothing better than nettle leaf; it is a valued remedy to alleviate itching and minimize histamine production in conditions of hives, food sensitivities, or allergic reactions. I find that it works best when it is consumed and ingested a month or so prior to expected allergy season.

- Use for removal of uric acid buildup in gout and for rheumatism and to relieve excess fluid and wastes from the body through the kidneys.
- **For hypertension:** combine with heart herbs for support.
- **As a lactation stimulant:** prepare an infusion with fennel and caraway.
- **For insect bites:** apply as a topical poultice.

Combine with red raspberry and red clover leaf and use as a tea for a couple of months as a building, cleansing tonic for teenage girls, both for the high iron content and for hormone regulation. Its astringent nature helps to regulate excessive bleeding and heavy menstrual cycles and, really all types of bleeding, both internal and external.

Nettle leaf helps to remove uric buildup from the joints, making it a useful plant for gout and arthritis; it acts as a cleanser for systemic inflammations and around the joints. As a diuretic and for kidney support, nettle leaf can remove excess fluid and can be combined with other antilithic herbs for kidney stones. It is thought that nettles work to both reduce levels of anti-inflammatory cytokines and may stimulate secretion of interleukin-6, decreasing prostaglandin synthesis and contributing to an anti-inflammatory effect.[234]

As a food, nettles are a delicious spring vegetable added into soups, egg dishes, and stews or it can be steamed as a side vegetable with butter, coconut oil, fresh lemon juice, and fresh herbs. Juice the fresh leaves, or freeze nettles and use for cooking in later months.

Nettles are safe and nontoxic; however, fresh stinging nettle leaf should not be consumed raw. Check out the fine hairs in the nettle picture on page 140. Drying or cooking the leaves inactivates the stinging hairs, making it safe for ingestion. Be sure to steam the leaves first before juicing. Avoid if one is sensitive to histamine or allergic to nettles.

## Clear Skin Relief

1 teaspoon dried Nettle leaf
1 teaspoon Red Clover leaf and flower
1 teaspoon Chickweed herb
1 teaspoon Cleavers herb

Prepare an infusion and ingest for acne and skin conditions.

## AllerBGone Tea

2 teaspoons dried Nettle leaf
1 teaspoon dried Plantain leaf
1 teaspoon dried Chamomile flowers
2 teaspoons dried Goldenrod leaf

Prepare as an infusion and consume frequently during the allergy season. The antiallergy flavonoid-rich components and antihistamine constituents will provide relief from congestion, sneezing, and itchy eyes.

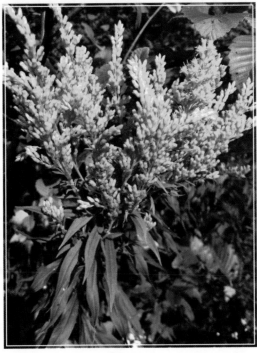

**Goldenrod: *Solidago spp.***

## Corn Silk Stigmas

I still remember my astonishment when I first discovered that the herb *Zea mays*, a.k.a. corn silk, was the husk of the very corn consumed as a food. It is one thing to learn of an herb through a textbook, but it is surprising to learn how many medicinal plants are ones which we see on a regular basis and are flourishing in our environment. I'm certain you have pulled open the husk and removed corn for cooking. The silk inside the corn husk is used either fresh or dried as an herbal medicine. It is known by herbalists as a demulcent of interest for the urinary tract, gently soothing irritation to the mucous membranes for stones in the urine, cystitis, and prostate inflammation when combined with other related herbs.

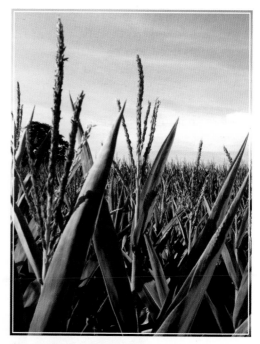

**Corn Silk Stigmas (*Zea mays, Stigmata maidis*) Family: *Poaceae***

Maize or corn is a valuable staple food in many cultures. As a medicine, the silky fine threads (styles and stigmas of female corn) are collected before pollination. They are generally a light brown, though are sometimes red or light green in color.

**Constituents:** saponins, allantoin, vitamin C, volatile alkaloids, phytosterols, tannin,[235] bitter glycosides, vitamin C, rutin, flavonoids, resins, fixed oil[236]

**Medicinal Action:** diuretic, anti-lithic, anti-inflammatory, weakly hypotensive, weak antiseptic, demulcent

**Applications:** infusion, tincture

Corn silk is a soothing demulcent herb for painful urination related to cystitis or a urinary tract infection, working well as an anti-irritant for excessive uric acid. Corn silk's demulcent effects gently soothe irritated mucous membranes lining the urinary tract. They are added to kidney tea blends to enhance the diuretic effect or combined with other antilithic herbs for stones in the kidneys or bladder.

Consider using this valuable herb for humans and animals alike. As herbal medicines, they can certainly be of assistance to our furry friends and barnyard animals.

It can also be combined with relaxant and heart tonic herbs such as hawthorn, yarrow, and lemon balm for assistance with an elevated blood pressure.

### Soothing Cystitis Corn Silk Tea
2 part Corn Silk stigma
1 part Plantain leaf
½ part Spearmint

Prepare as an infusion to alleviate painful voiding and urination.

## Mullein Flower and Leaf

Mullein has many names, from our lady's flannel to beggar's stalk to golden rod (not to be confused with *Solidago canadensis,* another herb). It is recognized by its downy soft leaves and one tall spiked stalk containing velvety yellow flowers (recognized by five petals) which grow in the second year. The downy hair on both sides of the leaves offers protection from grasshoppers and birds wanting to ingest the leaves—the fluff can be irritating if ingested by cattle. Mullein prefers dryer soils and can grow up to nine feet high in some areas. It is readily found on mountainsides and roadsides, in the Okanagan and the interior of BC; it is found in groves and on almost

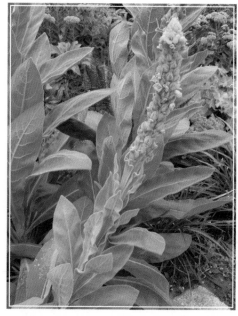

**Mullein Flower and Leaf (*Verbascum thapsus*) Family: *Scrophulariaceae***

every hillside.[237] Be sure to gather the leaves, flower, and stems in dry weather before they turn brown on the stalk—early summer until August is a good time. For those who enjoy camping, use the dried stalk and decomposing dried mullein leaves of fall as tinder to start a campfire.[238]

**Constituents of flower:** mucilage, flavinoids (rutin, hesperidin), saponins, tanning and volatile oil,[239] verbascoside

**Constituents of leaf:** mucilage, iridoids, saponins, flavonoids[240] Verbascoside and flavonoids contribute to the demulcent, anti-inflammatory, and emollient properties.

**Medicinal Actions:** demulcent, antitussive, expectorant, diaphoretic, astringent, sedative, soothing relaxant, mild antiseptic, diuretic, chest tonic, emollient, anti-inflammatory

**Applications:** infusion, smoke, poultice, ear oil, infused oil, tincture

The flowers offer both soothing mucilage, anti-cough properties, and expectorant abilities from its saponin constituents; reach for this herb for irritated respiratory passages. Traditionally, the dried leaves were blended into herbal smoking mixtures—today, mullein flowers and leaves are key expectorant agents for loosening ample, extensive phlegm in bronchial congestion, asthma, emphysema, and breathing difficulties. Used during a cold or flu, mullein has diaphoretic actions, promoting sweating to reduce a high temperature. Its antimicrobial properties can be used for a sore throat or infections of the urinary tract.

Prepare mullein infused oil as ear drops for an earache, the mumps, and middle ear infection. This infused oil can also nourish dry skin in the case of dry, scaling skin and eczema.

A warm mullein poultice can be applied for hemorrhoids and for pain relief associated with stiffness and arthritis. Known as a wound healer, mullein can be used topically as an anti-inflammatory agent to reduce swellings.

## Mullein Hemorrhoid Enema Infusion
1 teaspoon Mullein leaf and flower
1 teaspoon Self-heal herb
1 teaspoon Heartsease herb
1 teaspoon Red Raspberry leaf
1 teaspoon Chamomile flower
Enema bag

Prepare an infusion by using equal parts of all or any of these herbs. Prepare 2 cups of tea using 2 heaping tablespoons of herbs to 2 cups water. Steep for 15 minutes, creating a strong tea. Strain and cool until lukewarm, taking care not to burn. Pour into an enema bag, ensuring the tip is well lubricated, and use as a retention enema for 10 minutes. The astringent herbs will come in direct contact with the inflamed tissues, providing healing and reducing irritation and inflammation, while also providing antiseptic properties. Use daily for acute conditions until the condition resolves; take steps to ensure no constipation is present.

## Goldenrod

A bright and beckoning plant, goldenrod can be found alongside roadways when heading out of town and by the sides of meadows in the woods. Keep your eyes open for the sprays of golden wildflower tops and a plant growing up to six feet tall. The aerial plant parts—the fragrant flowers and leaves—are harvested in the summer when the plant has begun flowering. The leaves, roots, and flowers are used medicinally.

**Constituents:** flavonoids, (rutin, quercetin—a natural antihistamine), saponins, tannins[241]

**Medicinal Actions:** antiallergic, anticatarrhal, antifungal, carminative, anti-inflammatory, diuretic, kidney tonic, diaphoretic, antiseptic

**Applications:** infusion, herbal vinegar, salve, cream, powder, tincture, herb wash, honey

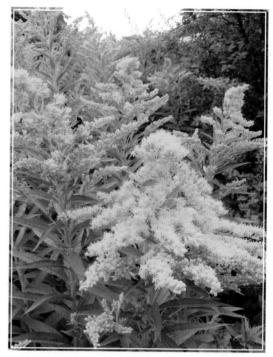

Goldenrod (*Solidago virgaurea* and *canadensis* – and other various species) **Family:** *Asteraceae*

Goldenrod is a spring tonic herb for use during the allergy season to help minimize excess production of mucous in the lungs and upper respiratory tract. It contains quercetin, an antihistamine, antiallergy flavonoid, which helps to decrease the production of allergic histamines in our bodies. For best results combine with nettle leaf.

A soothing anti-inflammatory, diuretic, and antiseptic herb ideal for urinary tract infections, combine with corn silk and plantain. Traditionally this herb was used for anuria (the absence of urine due to acute nephritis, an inflammation of the glomeruli in the kidneys) through a program of fasting and consuming a tea of goldenrod and parsley seed.[242] Although I recommend that for any chronic condition, it is best to be under the clinical care of a medical herbalist.

The antifungal properties are due to saponins, thus offering relief from athlete's foot, nail fungus, vaginal yeast infections, and oral candidiasis (thrush).[243]

Another go-to spit poultice, use the leaf for insect bites. A common term for this plant is woundwort, as the herb is used to stop the bleeding of wounds when used topically as a poultice.

- **For hemostatic actions:** use the leaf and prepare a poultice to stop bleeding of wounds.
- **For pain of arthritis and sciatica:** use as an anti-inflammatory poultice.
- **For sore throat and gum inflammation:** prepare an infusion and use as a throat gargle.
- **As a carminative and digestive aid:** prepare an infusion.
- **As a wound healer with anti-inflammatory properties:** apply topically.
- **As a diuretic and kidney tonic with anti-inflammatory properties:** use the tincture or infusion.
- **For relief of a toothache:** chew the leaf.

Herbalist Bev Gray, in her book *The Boreal Herbal,* suggests using goldenrod leaves as a substitute to spinach when gathered in the spring, sautéed or steamed and added into omelettes or soups.

## Goldenrod Styptic Powder
1 part Goldenrod herb
1 part Yarrow herb
½ part Cayenne pepper powder

Using a coffee grinder, blend all 3 herbs into a fine powder. Pour into a spice container. Keep in the first cabinet and apply directly onto open wounds as a styptic or hemostatic agent (it will stop bleeding and assist in blood coagulation). Apply the powder to open, bleeding wounds and thoroughly fill the area. Apply pressure and elevate wound until bleeding stops.

**Note:** Some individuals have allergies to the Daisy family of plants.

## Juniper

**Parts Used—Berries and Needles:** The berries turn a dark purple-blue when ripe (sometimes with a whitish film over the blue), taking two to three separate summers to mature, and increasing in sweetness as they age. Gather the berries in the fall, when ripe. The needles can be gathered at any time. If hiking, especially above the tree line, look for this low-lying shrub in sunny meadows with dark blue berries, sometimes tinged with white. The berries are used medicinally and can be dried and stored for future use in a glass container.

**Constituents:** volatile oils, vitamin C, flavonoids, resin, tannins[244]

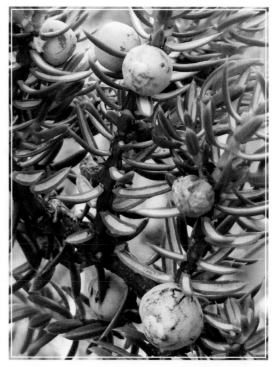

Juniper (*Juniperus communis* (Common Juniper) *Juniperus horizontalis* (Creeping Juniper)) Family: *Cupressaceae*

**Medicinal Actions:** alterative, analgesic, antibacterial, anti-inflammatory, antimicrobial, antirheumatic, antiseptic, aromatic, carminative, diaphoretic, digestive aid, diuretic, emmenagogue, rubefacient, tonic, urinary antiseptic, uterine stimulant

**Applications:** baths, infused oil, liniment, tincture, infusion, salve, massage oil, food, honey, essential oil

Mixologists may know Juniper for flavoring gin and other liquors. The berries are delicious—try chewing them to freshen bad breath or use them in cooking. I frequently graze on the berries while hiking and am drawn to their fragrance and spicy taste. Experiment: add the berries into soups and stews (** they are the secret ingredient in my homemade chili!). Consider adding the berries into homemade sauerkraut, herbal honey, and wild game meat dishes, or try it with cedar-planked salmon—delicious!

As a medicine, juniper berries are strongly antiseptic for urinary tract infections, urethritis, and cystitis, but are also of value for prostatitis. The berries are cleansing and can enhance the removal of kidney stones, uric acid buildup, and toxins via the kidneys; combine with a soothing, antispasmodic, demulcent herb such as plantain or corn silk in a tea.

Juniper offers anti-inflammatory properties for painful joints, arthritis, sore muscles, gout, and cramping. Topically the berries can be prepared as an infused oil, an ingredient in salve or liniment for sore joints, and a topical application to the skin for symptoms of neuralgia.

Juniper essential oil is also available for topical application. I love the scent, however, it is very strong and needs to be diluted in a salve or carrier oil—never take the essential oil internally. This plant needs to be used respectfully.

As a steam inhalation, the berries can be crushed slightly with a mortar and pestle before adding into boiling water to release the volatile oils. Use as a steam inhalation for congestion, related to a cold or allergies, or place the crushed berries in a warm Epsom salt bath and obtain the antispasmodic and muscle-relaxing properties for the whole body. This is ideal for the onset of a flu, when muscle aches and chills are apparent.

- Use as an antimicrobial and antibacterial for gram-positive infections or long-ranging infections
- **For gas and bloating and to strengthen digestion:** prepare a digestive tonic and warming tea.
- **Traditional cold and flu remedy:** mix with rose hips and lemon balm as an infusion.
- **For cellulitis, acne, and to stimulate circulation:** use a topical application.
- **For dandruff:** prepare a decoction of the berries for a scalp rinse.

**Cleansing and Ceremonial purposes:** Juniper boughs can be burned on a charcoal disc as incense, the smoke used for purification of a home. The branches of juniper can be burned, similar to smudging with sage, to purify and remove negativity from a room. Hold a clear intention in your mind while using the smoke of the juniper bough to cleanse a space. According to boreal herbalist Bev Gray, in her book *The Boreal Herbal: Wild Food and*

*Medicinal Plants of the North*, the First Nations people have used juniper berries as an emergency food source. With strong antiseptic properties, it may also be used to cleanse the auric fields or spirit.

Avoid during pregnancy or if suffering from kidney disease, as the volatile oils in juniper may be too strong for weak kidneys. Use short term and in moderation.

## Juniper Antispasmodic Oil
Juniper berries and needles
Grape-seed Oil
3–4 drops Wintergreen or Pine Essential Oil

Crush the dried berries and bruise the juniper needles using a mortar and pestle. Cover with a carrier oil—grape-seed oil is a good choice. Infuse for 4 hours on low temperature. Strain and add in wintergreen or pine essential oil: 3–4 drops per 100 ml of infused oil. Use as a massage oil to limber up stiff, tense muscles after a workout or a day of hiking.

## Juniper Cold Relief Tea
1 part Juniper berries, crushed
1 part Rose Hips
1 part Lemon balm leaves

Use equal portions of herbs to prepare an infusion. Steep 15 minutes, covered. Strain and drink 3–5 cups per day for flu-like symptoms, congestion, and elevated temperature at the onset of a cold. A warming, diaphoretic drink, this tea assists in lowering a fever while providing antiviral properties and immune-enhancing properties.

## Rose Hips and Wild Rose

Closer to home, the wild rose is the official emblem flower of Alberta, the province beside British Columbia, where I live and where wild roses can be found growing in abundance in the wild: alongside riverbanks, roadsides, and wooded areas beside clearings and forests. The fruits (also known as the fleshy rose hips), flowers, roots, and leaves offer potent medicine. The leaves and roots are har-

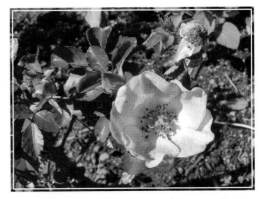

**Rose Hips and Wild Rose (*Rosa acicularis*) Family: *Rosaceae***

vested in the spring, the flowers in the summer. Rose petals can be collected in the morning once the dew has dried and before the heat of the midday sun. Harvest when the rose petals have nearly opened fully. Don't overharvest though: leave petals flowering on every bush to ensure pollination and propagation for future years. The fruit or rose hip is harvested in the autumn after the first frost from late August to mid-October, as the vitamin C content rises. The First Nations people consumed rose hips as a snack, picked and eaten right off the bush—but only the outer meat of the rose hip is eaten. If you have ever nibbled on a rose hip, you will find in the center some unpalatable furry seeds (don't eat them). Slit larger rose hips down half the side to remove the seeds. The hips can be dried and spread out on a cookie sheet—they will be crisp and brittle after a couple of days. Use the dried hips for tea or grind into a powder.

**Constituents:** Rose hips are rich in vitamin C, organic acids, carotenoids, flavonoids (quercetin, rutin), tannins[245]

**Medicinal Actions of fruits:** nutritive (vitamin c rich), anti-inflammatory, antiseptic, astringent, vermifuges, mild laxative, antimicrobial, diuretic, antispasmodic

**Medicinal Actions of flowers:** emollient, astringent, refrigerant, humectant

**Medicinal Actions of leaves:** astringent

**Applications for rose hips:** syrup, decoction, jam, jelly, nutritive food

**Applications for rose petals:** poultice for bites, eyewash, cosmetic, infused oil, infusion, tincture, salve, cream, essential oil, honey, vinegar

**Applications for leaves:** astringent poultice, gargle, tinctures

**Rose hips:** 100 g offers 426 mg of Vitamin C, 169 mg of Calcium, 1.06 mg of Iron, 69 mg of Magnesium, 429 mg of Potassium, 4345 IU of Vitamin A, and 5.84 mg of Vitamin E.[246] Use a dehydrator on low heat or air dry carefully to preserve the Vitamin C content. Take note of just how much Vitamin C 100 g of rose hips delivers: 426 mg of Vitamin C compared to a navel orange, where 100 g delivers 59.1 mg of Vitamin C (with 1 cup being 97.5 mg).[247] The vitamin content varies depending on time of collection, habitat, drying method, and species. Avoid collecting rose hips that have come in contact with sprays and pollution.

Rose hips are antioxidant-rich, containing flavonoids and quercetin. They are strengthening to the heart, capillaries, and connective tissue and are of benefit for varicose veins and hemorrhoids.

- **For hemorrhages, ulcers, and diarrhea:** use as an astringent.
  **For eye inflammation:** fresh, bruised petals prepared as a tea.
- Laxative, yet also used for diarrhea—balancing in nature.
- **Sore throat or tonsillitis:** rose syrup, infusion as a throat gargle.
- **Sachets:** dry rose petals to scent linen, spray or sprinkle homemade rosewater on linen.
- **Body care and cosmetic use:** for dry, mature skin—astringent to tighten pores.
- **Skin wash:** prepared as an infusion for ulcers, open wounds, and cuts
- The leaves contain tannins and bioflavonoids for diarrhea, and a gargle for a sore throat.
- **For cosmetic use and body care:** there is nothing more luscious than rose. Known as a humectant, similar to honey, it retains moisture on the skin. It can be used as an astringent wash for oily and problem skin, as well as nourishing for dry and delicate, aging skin. Prepare a facial steam as a skin tonic and finish by applying ice water to the face to close the pores. The infused oil of rose creates one of the finest massage oils delicately scented with rose.

## Rose Hip Syrup

Place 200 grams Rose hips in a pan (after topping and tailing) or cut in a food processor.

Cover with 750 milliliters of water, bring to boil, and simmer on low heat for 15 minutes.

Strain out liquid using a sieve or muslin, then repeat. Add the Rose hip pulp back into the pot with 500 ml more water. Simmer for an additional 15 minutes then strain. Mix the two juices together and reheat until boiling.

Add 150–200 grams Sugar or Maple syrup, or add in a bit of Brandy as a preservative.

Sweeten to taste, knowing that lower sugar will reduce the shelf life.

## Baby's Balm Rose Dusting Powder

1 teaspoon Rose petals, dried
1 teaspoon Lavender flowers, dried
1 teaspoon Chamomile flowers, dried
½ teaspoon Plantain leaf, dried
2 teaspoons Arrowroot powder

Blend ingredients, grinding in a mortar and pestle or coffee grinder, and add in arrowroot powder. Place in a glass spice container. Free from talc and cornstarch, use as a dusting powder for a baby's bottom after bathing to prevent chapping.

## Rose Water

Gather fragrant Rose petals and place in a glass or enamel pot. Cover with spring water and slowly bring to a boil. Simmer on low heat for 10 minutes and strain. Bottle.

Use as a hair rinse, in cooking, desserts, as a light perfume, for cosmetic use, or pour into a spritzer bottle and spray on linen to impart a fresh scent. To preserve the scent, add in 1 teaspoon of vodka as a fixative after bottling.

## Glycerine and Rosewater

5 parts Rose water (use recipe above)
2 parts Vegetable glycerine
½ part Witch Hazel

Rose and vegetable glycerine, being humectants, attract and retain moisture in the skin. I recall an herbal colleague and well-known local wild crafter, the late Nikaiah Jaguar, claiming that this was the very best nourishing solution for split, dry, cracked heels on the feet. So simple yet effective, this is a deliciously-scented remedy.

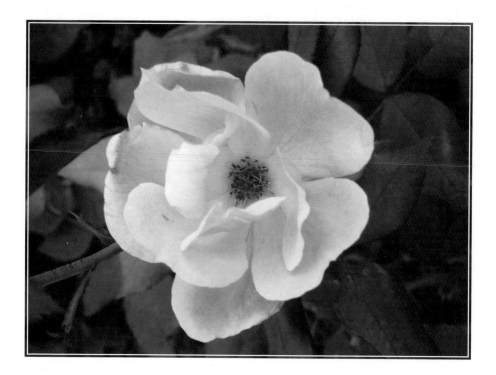

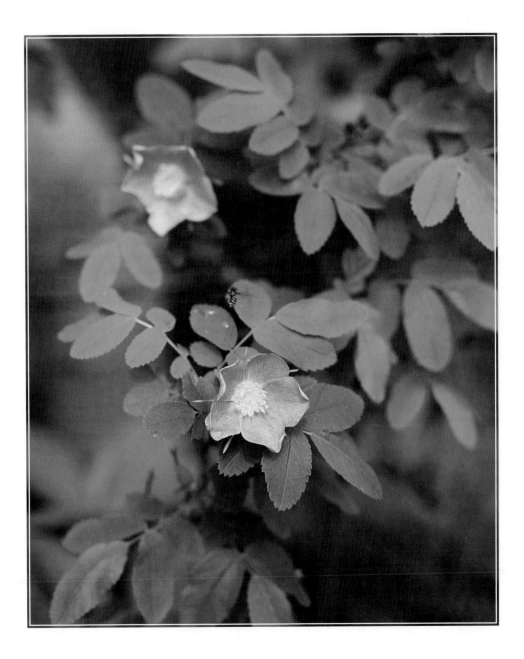

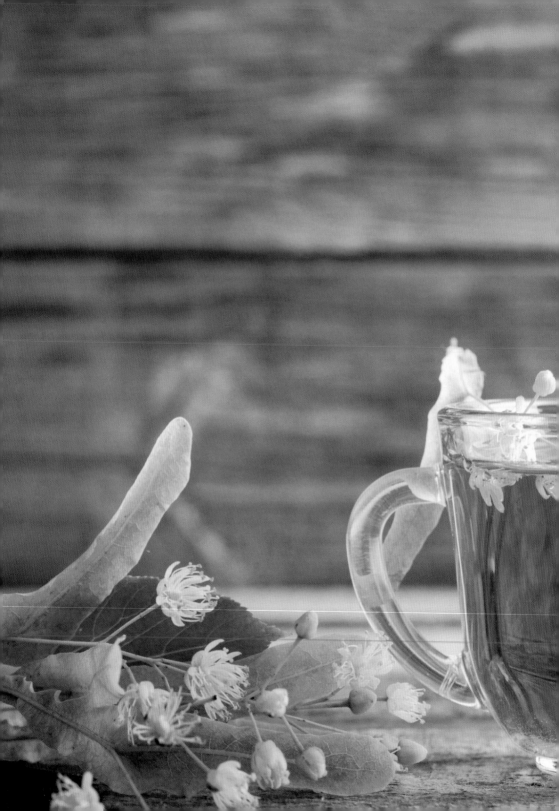

# PREPARING HERBAL REMEDIES: TECHNIQUES, TOOLS, AND RECIPES

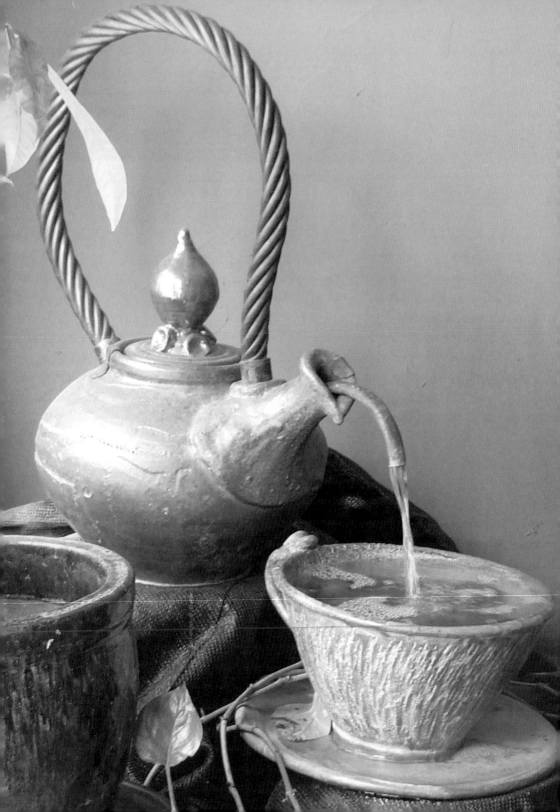

# Herbal Medicines and Treatments

## TEAS

For beginners, the first logical step of medicine-making is to prepare an herbal tea: a simple water-based preparation brewed either as an infusion or a decoction.

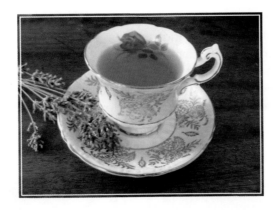

Enjoying conversation while sharing a cup of tea is a delightful way to spend an afternoon. It is an opportunity to align both with the plant and the desired outcome of the medicine. Tea time is an ideal opportunity to focus on one's intentions, practice gratitude, journal, write out desired outcomes, and visualize desired health goals.

### Infusions

If you brew Earl Grey tea, then you are creating an infusion. The process is straightforward. Simply boil water, pour over the herbs, cover, and then steep. Infusions are a process used for the more fragile parts of a plant, such as the flowers, leaves, fruit, and scented seeds. Infusions help retain the volatile oils of a plant; if preparing a tea for its high nutrition (mineral and vitamin) content, use an infusion. Think of infusions for delicate plant parts such as chamomile flowers, red clover blossoms, yarrow herb, thyme leaves, nettle leaf, cinnamon bark, and fennel seeds.

The Adult Dosage amount for medicinal teas involves using one heaping teaspoon of the dried plant for every cup of water, and drinking three to four cups of tea per day. This rule is, of course, variable depending upon the application, condition, and plants chosen. When using teas as medicine, remember that they are subtle—ensure that your ingestion and dosage is high enough to be effective.

### Tea Brewing 101

**Method 1:** Boil water on the stove. Place herbs in a container (ideally with a lid to contain the valuable volatile oils) and pour boiling water over herbs. Cover and steep 10-15 minutes. Pour the tea through a strainer while you inhale the volatile oils being released, and continue to inhale the scent while sipping.

**Method 2:** For a more concentrated tea, steep the tea overnight in a thermos or reheat on the stove in the morning. The tea will be potent medicine.

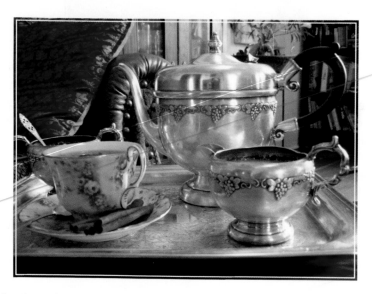

## Decoctions

Decoctions extract plant chemicals from harder, solid plant material such as roots, nuts, bark, and unscented seeds. There are a couple of exceptions. Some seeds and roots are high in volatile oils, which you can smell; examples are caraway seeds and valerian root, which are better infused to ensure that the volatile oils do not evaporate during the preparation process.

Three common decoction preparations exist.

**Method 1:** Add cold water to a pot on the stove and add in the herbs. Then bring the preparation up to a boil. Reduce the temperature and simmer on low heat, covered, for 15–20 minutes. Strain and drink.

**Method 2:** Boil water in a pot on the stove. Once boiling, reduce the heat to a low simmer, and add in the herbs. With the lid on, simmer for an additional 15–20 minutes.

**Method 3:** Overnight brewing is also possible for decoctions, again, creating stronger more potent medicine. For a stronger medicinal tea, decoct according to method 1 or 2 and let it sit overnight. It is possible that the plants can be reused again before discarding.

### Tips of the Craft
- When a tea has both hard nonaromatic roots and leaves, it is best to mix the plant parts separately. First prepare a decoction of the roots. Then remove from heat and add the leaves to infuse, covered, for an additional 15 minutes.
- Not all chemicals from herbs are extracted with just water: resins, lipids, and alkaloids, for example, require alcohol for complete extraction.
- Teas can be stored in the fridge for a couple days and reheated on the stove.
- Popular during warm summer months, drinking medicinal teas cold will provide a delicious cool drink but will increase the diuretic properties of a plant. So plan accordingly.

### Tisane Flavoring

Tea blending is a delightful art and the outcome is delicious medicine. The more tart, bitter plant parts can be easily masked by adding in tastier aromatic herbs. Some of my favorite flavorings include rose hips, stevia, chamomile, pineapple weed, fennel, spearmint, rose, lavender, caraway, spearmint, ginger, cinnamon, star anise, fennel, and lemon balm.

For children or individuals with fussy taste buds, dry or fresh herbs can be muddled and prepared as an infusion or decoction and then administered as a tea or mixed with fruit juice, but be mindful of the sugar content. For children, a tea mixture can be the start of a delicious frozen treat. To create freezer pops, blend in with fresh fruit and create frozen fruit/ herbsicles. Medicinal herbal teas can be added into a morning smoothie or disguised in a soup or stew.

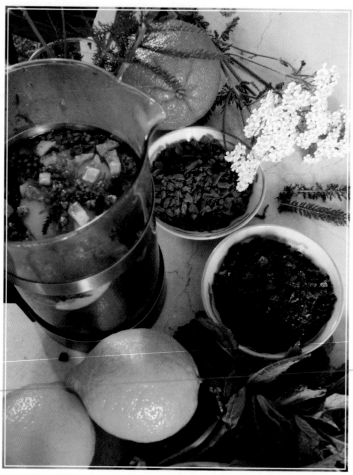

**Yarrow Rosehip Cold & Flu Relief Recipe (page 107)**

# Soothe My Throat Gargle

**Ingredients**
1 part Thyme herb or Rosemary
1 part Marigold flower
1 part Cleavers herb
½ part Salt
2 cups boiling water

**Directions**
Prepare an infusion of equal parts of the herbs or any one of the herbs above. Pour boiling water over the herbs and steep, covered, for 15 minutes. Strain, and stir in the salt. Gargle with warm tea until liquid is used completely. Repeat 2–3 times per day or hourly for acute conditions.

Too often a sore throat can be the beginning of a deeper immune assault. This potent blend containing volatile oils offers potent antiviral and antibacterial properties. Use for a sore throat; I use it after a day of teaching when my voice is often hoarse and sore. It works like a charm.

## STEAMING
Steaming is an ideal inhalation therapy for any ailment relating to the respiratory system, including colds, congestion, seasonal allergies, and lung infections. The antiseptic volatile oils assist in disinfecting the mucous membranes of the upper respiratory tract and stimulating the immune system. The volatile oils found in essential oils, fresh herbs, or dried herbs contain antiviral, antibacterial, and antimicrobial properties.

When using essential oils, remember they are very concentrated—only four to eight drops are needed for a steam in a basin of hot water. Add the drops of essential oils into boiling water and steam immediately; the volatile oils will slowly evaporate under the high heat. Place your head under a tea towel and inhale the steam for several minutes to open up the sinus passages.

**Steaming with dried herbs:** Use 3–4 teaspoons of herbs per 4 cups of boiling water. Cover and steep for at least 5 minutes before steaming, with your head under the towel.

Fresh herbs require more plant material; use about 5–6 tablespoons of chopped fresh plants per 4 cups boiling water.

** Remember, steam is hot! Take care not to burn sensitive mucous membranes. For small children, test the heat of the steam first before using for a youngster to prevent burning.

# Sinus Relief Herbal Steam

## Ingredients
1 teaspoon dried Chamomile flowers
1 teaspoon dried Rosemary leaf
1 teaspoon dried Spearmint leaf
4 drops Eucalyptus Essential Oil

## Directions
Boil water, pour into a basin, and add the herbs. Steep, covered, at least 5 minutes. When ready to use, add the essential oil. Be mindful not to burn yourself with the hot bowl or the hot steam. Put your head under a tea towel to trap the steam and inhale the vapors. You will feel immediate relief as the steam and disinfectant volatile oils open up the sinus passages. For children, place a towel around the bottom of the bowl to protect from burning. Always try out the heat from the steam first, by putting your wrist under the towel before putting a young child, with sensitive tissues, in direct contact with hot steam.

## Herbal Baths
Herbal baths are similar to an herbal tea but are brewed into a larger vessel, such as a bathtub, for the whole body as a topical application. Use larger amounts of plant material and steep. Purchase a large cotton bag, or use some creativity—a clean cotton sock will work. It can be an effective tool for brewing tea in the bathtub. Using a bag keeps those tea bits from getting caught in the plumbing. Alternatively, purchase a stainless steel strainer to fit into the drain and simply brew the herbs loose.

If whole body applications, such as an herbal bath are not possible, then the wool sock treatment can be applied. Soak clean cotton socks in an infusion or decoction of warm herbal tea. Wring out and pull over the feet — place dry thick wool socks on overtop and head straight to bed. The heat of the wool will encourage absorption of the herbs through the delicate skin on the arches of the feet. This application works well for infants, young children, the elderly, and people who are unable to swallow medicine.

**Method 1:** Infuse or decoct 2–3 liters of herbal tea and steep in the bath water as a strong tea and use a strainer to catch the tea bits before they enter the plumbing.

**Method 2:** Fill a muslin or cotton bag with herbs, close the top, and suspend under the tap while running the bath water. An infused tea will be created in the bath as the water flows through the bag.

**Method 3:** Allow the closed cotton bag filled with herbs to soak in the bath.

A couple drops of essential oil of your choice can also be added into the bath water for added relaxant properties.

# RELAXATION BATH

## Ingredients
1 part Chamomile flowers
1 part Rose petals
1 part Lavender flowers
5 Cardamom seeds

## Directions
This exotic mixture is a reminder of ancient times when bathing was a ritual for health purposes. Blend ingredients together and place in a cotton sachet or bag. Hang over the flow of water from the bath and infuse. Or scatter freely in the bath and place a metal drain strainer to catch water-soaked petals after the bath has been enjoyed.

**Muscle Relaxing:** Ginger, Turmeric, Chamomile, Eucalyptus
**Sleep Promoting:** Lavender, Chamomile, Lemon Balm, Pineapple weed
**Energizing Baths:** Rosemary, Basil, Peppermint, Spearmint
**Diaphoretic Herbs for Colds and Flu:** Yarrow, Peppermint, Ginger, Sage, Thyme, Oregano, Eucalyptus

Tea, baths, poultices, and fomentations can all be prepared using either fresh or dried herbs macerated in hot water. Where one part dried herb is called for, use three parts more fresh herb due to the moisture content of the fresh plant material.

## POULTICES
Created from essentially an herbal tea, the application of a poultice varies. A poultice involves the application of herbs directly onto the skin. This is where the plant material in tea making would normally be discarded or (hopefully) composted. To prepare a poultice, add just enough liquid to macerate the herb, wring out the plant from the liquid until almost dry, and then this moist herb mixture is applied directly to the skin.

## Applications for Poultices and Fomentations

- Tissue restorative for skin lacerations and abscesses.
- Pull out infections for eruptions, boils, lesions.
- Relief of inflammations: arthritis, swellings, gout.
- Stimulate circulation by supplying a rubefacient effect and improved blood flow to an area.
- Stop bleeding.
- Assist in sealing wounds.
- Pull out venom, splinters, and agents embedded in the skin.
- Assist to improve organ function.
- Relief of swollen glands, mumps, and blockages.
- Relief of sinus and chest infection for colds, allergies, asthma, bronchitis.

**Poultice Preparation:** Finely break up, chop, grind, or bruise the leaves using a mortar and pestle or blender. Add just enough moisture (hot water or herbal tea for a more medicinal blend) to make a thick paste; the herbs can be mixed with plantain or ground flaxseed for additional pulling power. First wash the skin with chamomile or calendula tea or tincture as a disinfectant. Then cover the skin with a thin layer of vegetable oil (grape-seed oil, or olive oil) as a protective barrier (to prevent blistering) and to enhance the penetration of the plant actives through the skin. Apply poultice herbs directly to the skin or wrap the paste in a wet, hot cloth (cheesecloth, a towel, or an old clean sweatshirt or sheet). Cover with plastic wrap to retain heat. For a poultice to be effective, it must be kept warm and moist. Use a hot pack or hot water bottle to retain heat; repeat for the second application. After removing the poultice, wash the area with herbal tea or antiseptic tinctures again to further healing.

**Note:** Mustard or onion poultices require a thin application of oil as protection for the skin. Prevent direct contact with the skin by keeping the paste buffered between two pieces of cloth. A necessity for an infant, monitor temperatures to prevent burning or blistering.

## Pineapple Weed Plantain Poultice

Prepare this poultice for wound healing and relief of insect bites and burns, even drawing out foreign objects like slivers embedded in the tissues. Prepare enough herbs to cover the affected area. Blend, grind, or even chew the fresh plants. Add hot water or oil to create a thick paste. Apply four times daily or as needed until the irritation resolves. Dried herbs can also be used.

## FOMENTATIONS

A fomentation uses flannel or fabric soaked in the tea liquid. Strain the herbs (or apply the herbs first as a poultice) then use the remaining liquid to soak a cloth. Wring out and apply the cloth to the body. Fomentations are often used for awkward body parts, such as the wrist, elbow and knee. Then apply heat (a hot water bottle, rice pack, or heating pad).

For a more potent decoction, soak the herbs in apple cider vinegar, adding in a small amount of cayenne powder or ginger to encourage more circulation and warmth to the area. Compresses made with vinegar will offer assistance from persistent tight muscles, aches, and joint pain.

### Fomentation Preparation

1. Prepare an infusion, decoction, or steep herbs in apple cider vinegar, using 1 part herb to 3 parts liquid. Steep 15–20 minutes, covered; the goal is a very concentrated tea. Strain the tea and keep warm for reapplication.
2. Soak a thick cloth in the hot tea (consider a cut cotton sheet, wool, linen, a kitchen tea towel, clean sweatshirt, or even a diaper—being creative will ensure the desired outcome).
3. Squeeze the cloth so it is barely damp.
4. Feel the cloth to test how hot it is. The goal is a hot temperature without burning the skin.
5. Secure over desired location and apply heat to the area.
6. When temperature drops, re-soak cloth and repeat.

**Remember:**

- The fomentation should be wrung out so it is barely damp with no fluid running out of the compress
- Large enough application to cover the area needing treatment
- Keep damp and hot as possible
- Repeat 3–4 times a day

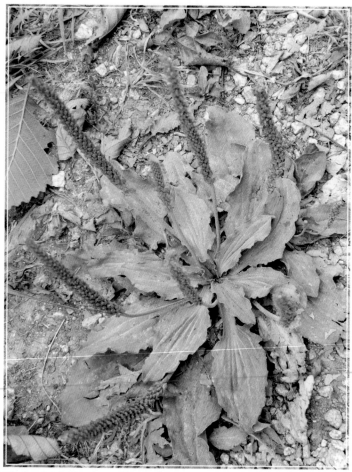

**Plantain (*Plantago major*)**

# MULLEIN GINGER FOMENTATION

Ideal for cramping or intestinal, menstrual, or muscular spasms, and for clearing sinus congestion, bronchitis, or spastic coughs.

**Ingredients**
1 cup fresh, grated Ginger root
1 teaspoon dried Mullein or Plantain leaf
2 teaspoons dried Eucalyptus leaves
½ teaspoon Cayenne pepper powder
2 liters distilled water

**Directions**
Boil fresh ginger in water on the stove for 10–15 minutes. Remove from heat, and add in mullein, eucalyptus, and cayenne. Steep an additional 15 minutes. Strain. Follow the preparation steps above for topical application.

# Herbal Vinegars

Herbal vinegars are slightly more potent than herbal teas; the vinegar can be used to pull out more plant constituents than simply using water alone. Proportions vary depending upon the bulkiness of the fresh or dried plant matter being used—a 1:2 ratio up to 1:5 ratio is a guide. One part plant matter to two parts vinegar can be used. Ensure that the herbs are completely covered with 1-2 inches more vinegar above the plants. Some dried plant material is extremely "thirsty" and after an hour or a day, the menstruum may appear to disappear, getting soaked into the plant. Add in extra vinegar to even out this balance. Fresh or dried plant material can be used, keeping in mind the need for more vinegar with fresh herbs (due to more moisture in fresh plants). Therefore, use a higher amount of vinegar, 1:5, to ensure shelf life.

## Ingredients
1 part fresh or dried Herbs
2 parts (to up to 5 parts) Apple Cider Vinegar

## Directions
If using fresh herbs, wash and pat dry, removing mangled or bug-munched leaves. Chop finely or mince to increase the surface area of the plant coming into contact with the menstruum. Place herbs in a container and fill with vinegar. Ensure the plant matter is covered with 2 inches of additional vinegar. Within 24 hours, if the menstruum is below the herbs, then top up with extra vinegar, covering another 2 inches above the herbs. Cover and place out of direct sunlight. Shake daily and infuse for 2—4 weeks. Strain. Store the vinegar in the fridge for 4—6 months; I find that my bottles are empty far sooner than that. Use the vinegar in a salad or drizzled over steamed vegetables.

## TIPS

For a nice visual touch, add in fresh or dried herb sprigs, flowers, peppercorns, chili peppers, and even berries as optional colorful additions, depending upon the flavor and base of the vinegar.

For those passionate about culinary creations, white or rice wine vinegar can also be chosen for variation, but apple cider vinegar has the highest health benefits.

Although I have never encountered this, if there is any mold, continued fermentation, or bubbles, then something has gone sideways. Discard and start again adding in more vinegar. Avoid the use of metal containers for vinegars—that is a chemical reaction just waiting to happen.

Savory flavors blend well together, as do mints with berries. Herb choices can be medicinal and still taste great. Herbal vinegars are great choices for mineral-rich plants.

Some great options for herbal vinegars include:

- anise
- basil
- caraway
- fennel
- garlic
- ginger
- lemon balm
- nettles
- oregano
- red clover
- rose
- rosemary
- spearmint

# LEMON BASIL VINEGAR

## Ingredients
4 teaspoons dried Basil leaves
3 teaspoons dried Lemon balm leaves
2 tablespoons fresh grated Orange peel
½ teaspoon dried Caraway seed
2 cups Apple Cider Vinegar

## Directions
Steep 2–3 weeks. Strain and rebottle. Use as a digestive agent diluted in water and drink prior to meals, or use as a salad dressing, mixing with olive oil and fresh lemon. Keep cool.

# Mineral-Rich Mix

**Ingredients**
1 part Red Clover leaf and flower
1 part Nettle leaf
1 part Chickweed herb
1 part Lemon Balm leaf
1 part Dandelion leaf
Apple Cider Vinegar to cover

**Directions**
Cover herbs with apple cider vinegar and steep 2–4 weeks. In my experience the leafy greens soften up and do not need straining, but of course follow your own preference.

# WINTER ANTIMICROBIAL VINEGAR

## Ingredients
2 parts fresh Onion, chopped
2 cloves Garlic, chopped
3 parts dried Rosemary leaf
3 parts dried Mullein leaf or flower
3 parts dried Yarrow leaf or flower
2 parts Juniper berries, fresh or dried
½ part dried Cinnamon root
½ part dried Clove fruit
1/5 part Cayenne—just a pinch
Honey
Apple Cider Vinegar to cover

## Directions
Fill into a glass jar. Cover with an additional inch of vinegar. Add enough apple cider vinegar to cover and steep 2–3 weeks, then strain. Take 2–3 times on a teaspoon at the onset of a cold, flu, and for symptoms of a sore throat. Add in honey for taste and for its preservative properties. Use as a salad dressing, take off the spoon, or use to season vegetables.

### The Lowdown on Apple Cider Vinegar

Apple cider vinegar is an ancient folk remedy used by generations of herbalists for numerous health issues. Created through a fermentation process, apple cider vinegar contains minerals, primarily potassium, magnesium, acetic and citric acid. Choose an unpasteurized, unfiltered apple cider vinegar containing the live nutrients, enzymes, and beneficial fermented bacteria called a scoby or mother. The "Mother" is a desired slimy or stringy mass found in unpasteurized products indicating that the active properties are still present in the vinegar.

## Folk Medicine Use of Apple Cider Vinegar

- Digestive aid, increasing hydrochloric acid in the stomach and sterilizing its contents, wards off foreign bacteria.
- May assist to lower fluid retention and hypertension.
- Helpful for rheumatism, leg cramps, and eliminating uric acid buildup.
- A home remedy for migraines and tension headaches.
- A useful addition to a cleanse or detox program.
- Gargle for relief from symptoms of a sore throat.
- Ingest for sinus congestion and cold and flu prevention (mixed with honey and cayenne).
- A topical application diluted in water for poison ivy, sunburn, skin rashes, warts, shingles, insect bites.
- Diluted in water and ingested before bed may help to lower blood sugar levels in the morning.
- Skin toner: Wash the face with apple cider vinegar (diluted in water and used as a rinse), this helps change the PH of the skin, warding off bacterial infection.
- Apple cider vinegar mixed with horseradish is a traditional home remedy for fading dark spots on the face—paint the spot daily.
- Natural deodorant: Soak moistened cotton pads and apply to the underarm and also to the feet. The vinegar smell will dissipate when dried and the antifungal and antibacterial agents will be a welcome relief for smelly feet and body odor.
- Dilute in water and use as a scalp and hair rinse for removing shampoo buildup, dandruff and for healthy shiny hair.

## TINCTURES

Tinctures are a way of soaking plants in a suitable solvent, generally a proportion of water and alcohol. Alcohol is the best solvent to extract chemical constituents from the plants and provides the longest shelf life of any preparation.

Herbalists most refer to alcohol and water-based preparations as "tinctures," but they can also mean products made with apple cider vinegar or vegetable glycerine. While not as strong, vinegar of glycerine can be considered for those with alcohol sensitivities, young children, those with liver issues, and/or those on numerous medications, or those avoiding alcohol for religious reasons or pregnancy.

Tinctures can be prepared using dried or fresh plant matter. When using fresh herbs, one needs to take into consideration the amount of moisture already contained in the fresh plant material in order to ensure a long shelf life and prevent spoilage. When making tinctures at home, gin, brandy, or vodka (or Everclear, if accessible) may be used as a menstruum.

The simplest tincturing process is the Traditional Folk Method:

1. Select your herbs of choice—fresh or dried plant material is just fine—and chop or shred finely. Do not use powdered.
2. Place herbs in a clean glass jar with a secure lid and a neck large enough to fit your hand for ease of cleaning.
3. Pour vodka over the herbs to cover entirely, adding 2 inches more above the plant material, as the herbs should be completely covered.
4. Secure the lid and shake daily; use this time to infuse the herbs with intention.
5. Soak 4 to 6 weeks, strain, and use your medicine.

Adult dosage of most tinctures: 3–5 ml taken 3 times daily, diluted in hot water, and taken before meals.

# Happy Tummy Aperitif

## Ingredients
1 part Yarrow herb
1 part Peppermint herb
½ part Sage herb
½ part Fennel seed

## Directions
Place herbs in a wide-mouthed jar and cover with alcohol. Ensure that the liquid covers the herbs about an inch higher than the herbs themselves. Place the lid on securely. Shake daily for 2 weeks. Strain and dilute 1 teaspoon in 1 ounce of water and sip prior to meals as a digestive aid and appetite stimulant.

*If using fresh herbs, chop the aerial plant parts to increase the surface area coming in contact with the menstruum. Fill with vodka, about 2 inches higher than the volume of fresh plants.

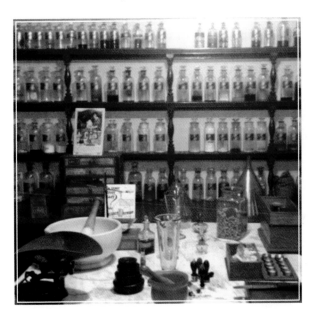

# HERBAL SYRUPS

Syrups are effective cough medicine and a tasty way for children (and adults alike) to take herbal medicine for a variety of ailments, including colds, digestion, and a sore throat. Delicious herbal syrups can also be used as ingredients in cocktail mixology and drink recipes. They can be drizzled over fruit or a baked desert; or add into a tea or tincture for flavor and secondary medicinal support.

## SYRUP MAKING

Simmer herbs in water on the stove as a decoction (or sometimes an infusion), reducing the fluid mixture to about half the concentration. Strain. Measure the volume of the liquid and add in an equal amount of sweetener. Warm the mixture over low to medium heat to thicken the syrup, stirring to prevent burning. Remove from heat. Cool and bottle. Store in the refrigerator for up to 8 weeks. Brandy can be added for its warming, spicy flavor, its anti-cough properties, and to extend the shelf life. Additional flavorings include: a fruit concentrate, orange or lemon peel, or a couple of drops of aromatic essential oil, such as peppermint or spearmint.

The sweet base (maple syrup or honey) creates a palatable medicine that can be taken off the spoon. Traditionally white sugar was used to prevent mold or yeast from forming at a 2:1 ratio of sweetener to liquid. However, if it is too sweet for your palate, reduce the amount of sweetener and be prepared for a shorter shelf life. I personally prefer a 1:1 ratio of sweetener.

| Syrup Ingredients to Prevent Fermentation |
| --- |
| Honey |
| Cane Sugar |
| Maple Syrup |
| Vegetable Glycerine |
| Black Cherry Syrup |
| Brandy |
| Orange or Lemon Peel |
| Brown Sugar |

# Sage Cherry Cough Syrup

A fantastic expectorant for spastic coughs, this formula can be taken for colds and flu, bronchitis, and pneumonia.

### Ingredients
2 teaspoons Sage leaf
2 teaspoons Mullein leaf or flower
2 teaspoons Plantain leaf
½ teaspoon Fennel seed
1 teaspoon Ginger root
4 cups Water
Brandy
⅓ cup Black Cherry concentrate
Honey or Sugar

### Directions
Place the herbs in the boiling water, reduce heat, and simmer covered for 20–30 minutes until the mixture is reduced to about half the volume. Set aside the heat and infuse for an additional 10 minutes, covered. Strain, measure, and add an equal volume (1:1 ratio) of honey to the tea. Mix in black cherry concentrate. Brandy can be added in as a preservative and also for flavor.

# HERBAL HONEYS

Pure, unpasteurized local honey has health benefits galore; a soothing cough syrup and antiseptic used internally and for purulent skin ulcers, burns, and infected open wounds externally. Combining honey with medicinal herbs creates delicious medicines! The possibilities are numerous and creativity plays a role in the endless possibilities, as do your taste buds.

Consider combining sage, rosemary, and fennel—a great remedy for sore throats.

Mix chamomile, lemon balm, and ginger to help with gas and bloating or an upset tummy.

Lavender, cinnamon, and basil work well together, as does my long time favorite for desserts: cinnamon, rose, and cardamom (just add a couple of cardamom seeds though, as they are potent).

*"My son, eat thou honey, for it is good."* —Proverbs 24:13

Amazing for children and adults alike, herbal honeys can be taken right off the spoon for minimizing spastic coughs, diarrhea, and of course the constant pain of sore throat. Add medicinal honeys to your tea blend, or drizzle over oatmeal and hot cereal or salads. Substitute honey where sweeteners are needed in a recipe—it can even be used to sweeten the tartest-tasting tincture. Consider using savory flavors over roasted vegetables and spicy or sweet flavors over fresh fruit, sorbets, coconut ice cream, and pies—the options are limitless. Herbal honeys can also be used as antiseptics topically, to aid in healing open wounds or added into body care products. While not as potent as a tincture, herbal honeys do offer medicinal benefit.

## HERBAL HONEYS

Fill a canning jar or wide open-mouthed container full with fresh herbs or ¼ full of dried herbs. Drizzle honey over the herbs to cover entirely. The honey should have lots of room to move around the herbs, so don't over pack the plants. Cap with a tight-fitting lid. Place in the sun and shake. Turn the jar over once a day or open up and stir to mix the plants with the honey. Sometimes herbs will swell or soak up the liquid when they are macerating. In this case, add in more honey to ensure the plants are entirely submersed. Infuse for 2–4 weeks. The therapeutic properties of the plants will be pulled out into the honey. Use the test of taste to determine the desired maceration time.

I like to leave the herbs in the honey, but if dried herbs are overly crunchy and hard (like cardamom or a woody bark), then it should be strained. If planning to remove the plant material, let your honey sit longer, like 3–4 weeks, before straining through a sieve for a stronger flavor. You can save these honeyed herbs and prepare tea from this sweet mixture. Should the honey harden before straining out the plant matter, then gently submerse the container in warm water to soften the honey. In order to preserve the nutrients and enzymes, don't overheat.

Herbs can be fresh or dried; both have their benefits. Fresh herbs contain a high water content, so the end result is a more watery solution with a shorter shelf life.

** There is certainly mixed opinion about serving honey to youngsters due to the rare risk of botulism spores, leading to chronic loose bowel movements in infants, possibly even death. Honey is a long-known antiseptic, so this could likely be another example of man-made opportunistic conditions. The presence of pesticide sprays and herbicides on flowers, and the act of pasteurization, kills the naturally-occurring antiseptic properties normally contained in honey. Individuals have used honey throughout the ages and not had an issue. However, based on the current state of things and to be safe, it is advisable not to feed honey to infants under the age of twelve months.

## ANTIMICROBIAL MANUKA HONEY

This honey is obtained by honeybees collecting pollen from the flowering manuka tree (*Leptospermum scoparium*) found growing in New Zealand and Australia. Manuka is one of the most potent therapeutic honeys, as it contains antibacterial and antifungal properties suppressing microbial growth. It is a known treatment for fighting infection, used in hospitals and wound care facilities for treating open wounds, for conditions of antibiotic-resistant infection, cellulitis, skin ulcers, purulent infections, and for treating burns. Honey has shown to be antimicrobial against staph, bacterial cellulitis, and antibiotic resistant infections such as *Bacillus subtilis*, methicillin-resistant *Staphylococcus aureus*,[248] *Escherichia coli*, ciprofloxacin-resistant *Pseudomonas aeruginosa*, and vancomycin-resistant *Enterococcus faecium*.[249]

In 2010, scientists at the University of Amsterdam reported that one of the manuka honey's antibacterial properties is from a protein called defensin-1.[250] The antibacterial and antimicrobial properties in honey arise from an enzyme reaction of glucose oxidase producing hydrogen peroxide.[251]

## HONEY HEALS

Skin Moisturizer: Honey is known as a humectant, meaning it holds in moisture, even drawing moisture from the air. Therefore it can help prevent scarring by keeping skin moist, preventing infection, and encouraging the growth of new tissues. Apply honey to a dressing to prevent it from sticking to the skin. Honey is a welcome addition to body care and hair care recipes alike: use as a moisturizer for dry scalp, seborrheic dermatitis, itching, and for reducing hair loss.

The World Health Organization (WHO) lists honey as a demulcent, a soothing substance that coats irritated mucous membranes, providing relief for a sore throat and spastic cough.[252]

**Note:** Each teaspoon of honey has nearly four grams of fructose, which means it should not be ingested for those who are diabetic, overweight, or fighting a Candida infection. If your health is good, then consuming raw honey, particularly herbal honeys in moderation, will offer health benefits. And remember to avoid the use of honey mixtures when camping in the forest!

## INFUSED OILS

The quality of the infused oils depends upon of the quality of the herbs and the carrier oil chosen. Grape-seed oil is the oil of choice due to its light quality, lack of scent and because it's readily available at a low cost. Almond oil, apricot kernel oil, even extra virgin olive oil are all excellent choices and can be

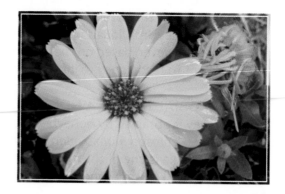

added into lotions, creams, massage oils, and of course the base for herbal infused oils. Use dried plant matter for infused oils with a couple of exceptions: St. John's Wort oil and Mullein flowers seem to tolerate fresh flower oil infusions without going moldy. For chamomile, rose, plantain, and all other infused oils, prepare using dried herbs to ensure longer shelf life and to minimize the risk of moisture, bacteria, and mold from entering the oil.

Preparation is simple. To prepare an infused oil, place the dry herbs in a Crock-pot or double boiler. Pour enough oil overtop to *completely* cover the herbs, with another inch or two of oil added to ensure complete covering. For those wanting exact measurements, standard proportions are a 1:8 to 1:10, so 1 part plant matter to 8 parts oil. If one part is 100 grams, then use 800 ml of oil.

Infused oils can be macerated in the sun. Place herbs and oil in a glass jar. Cover tightly and set in direct sun for 2 weeks, shaking daily. Strain the plant matter out of the oil, using a stainless steel strainer, cheesecloth, or a wine press for larger volumes, and rebottle. Store in a cool cupboard for a shelf life of about 8–12 months.

Crock-pots are a favorite for high-quality infused oils. Select one with 3 temperature settings. In my experience the hot setting is simply too hot—it can boil the oil. Medium is just right: a slow, steady heat to maintain the medicinal properties of the plants. Infuse for 2–4 hours for most herbs. Strain and rebottle. If no Crock-pot is handy, then prepare in a double boiler on the stove, ensuring that the mixture is on low temperature and never boils.

# Opulent Rose Body Oil

**Ingredients**
20 grams dried Rose flowers
20 grams dried Chamomile flowers
20 grams dried Lavender flowers
250–300 ml (approx.) Grape-seed Oil
10 ml Coconut Oil
5 drops Rose Essential Oil
20 drops natural Vitamin E Oil

**Directions**
Infuse flowers in grape-seed oil for 3–4 hours. Strain and mix in coconut oil while still slightly warm. Cool completely and add essential oil and vitamin E. Strain and rebottle. Works as a fabulous massage oil or use as a base for an herbal salve.

## HERBAL SALVES

Once you have prepared an herbal infused oil then you are just one simple step away from the creation of a salve—just add beeswax! Traditionally, simple salves were prepared using only oil or lard and beeswax, which provides the firmness to the salve. The medicinal properties can be enhanced by adding specific herbs into the infused oil or by choosing specific essential oils and/or tinctures. Transdermal absorption through the skin will occur as long as the skin is kept warm and moist; thus oil-based salves are more effective with longer absorption time than water-based creams.

## Basic Salve Recipe

Decide on the type of salve you are creating and for what outcome. Then prepare an herbal infused oil following one of the above methods. Strain the herbal oil and compost the plants. Place the oil in a double boiler on the stove. For each cup of herbal-infused oil, add $1/3$ to ¼ cup of beeswax, roughly (so a ratio of 1 part beeswax to about 3 parts to 4 parts oil, depending upon how hard one desires the salve). The best plan is to use the touch test! Heat the oil and beeswax together over low heat until the wax is completely melted. Add in just a small amount of beeswax at first; check for proper firmness by placing one drop of the oil on your finger and let it harden. Take your finger and test this consistency. If you desire a firmer salve, or you reside in a hot climate add more beeswax, or add more oil for a softer salve. The oil drop on your finger should be firm and not sticky or runny. The amount of beeswax needed will vary depending upon your

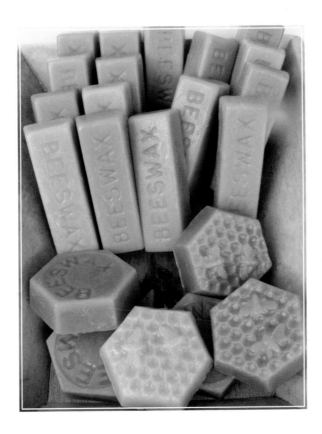

residence, the time of year, temperature, humidity, and ingredients used. When you are satisfied with the consistency, remove the salve mixture from the heat and use a ladle to scoop into small glass jars. Cool down to room temperature before securing the lids to ensure that no moisture is trapped in the container. Stored properly, a salve will last for months up to a year.

To extend the shelf life, a natural preservative like Vitamin E, a tincture of benzoin, or a couple drops of friar's balsam can be added into the salve before placing into jars.

If adding in tinctures or essential oils, whisk in the drops right before bottling as to prevent the heat from evaporating the properties.

# Chickweed Chamomile Salve

## Ingredients
$1/3$ cup Chickweed herbs, dried
$1/3$ cup Chamomile flowers, dried

Prepare an infused oil of the flowers above using 1½ cups of grape-seed oil and infuse using the recipe on page 233. Strain and use as salve base.
10 drops Marigold tincture
5 drops Lavender Essential Oil
Beeswax

## Directions
Pour the infused oil into a double boiler; grate beeswax and add into the infused oil. Once a small amount of beeswax has melted, test the consistency by placing one drop of the oil mixture on your hand, wait until it hardens, and determine if this is the desired consistency for your salve. If not, then add in a little more beeswax until you reach the desired amount. Take off the heat and quickly, before the salve hardens, whisk in 10 drops of Marigold tincture and 10 drops of lavender essential oil. Using a ladle, pour into containers and allow to cool fully before twisting the lid on the jar.

# MULLEIN AND GARLIC EAR OIL

## Ingredients
5 grams dried Mullein flowers
5 grams dried Self-heal flowers or herb
2 cloves of Garlic, peeled and finely minced

Cover with 50 ml Olive Oil and let sit for 3 days.
Strain and add in 4 drops of Tea Tree Essential Oil.

## Directions
Use drop dosages into the ear for middle ear infections, ear glue, or cold and flu symptoms.

## EAR OIL
Ear oils are applied by drop dosages to the ear canal and are effective for middle ear afflictions, symptoms related to a cold or flu, respiratory infections, mumps, ear glue, or infections. The blend offers antimicrobial and anti-inflammatory herbs to reduce swelling and pain, clear up infections, and moisten impacted ear wax in the ear canal.

# PLANTAIN MARIGOLD EYE BATH

## Ingredients
1 part Plantain leaf
1 part Marigold flower
1 part Pineapple Weed herb

## Directions
Prepare a strong infusion using distilled water. Steep for 15 minutes. Strain through a coffee filter to ensure there are no flower bits left in the wash. Pour into an eyecup and bathe each eye while mixture is warm, opening and closing the eye before discarding the solution. Repeat.

## EYE BATHS
Eyewashes are effective for inflammations, minor irritations, and allergies. Clean the eye cup to ensure it is sterile and use the infusion immediately after preparation, while still warm. Numerous soothing astringent herbs can be infused or the tincture used, diluted in hot water.

# FOR THE BODY

## ROUTINES AND TECHNIQUES
### Skin Brushing
Vibrant, glowing skin is the sign of a healthy body. As we age, our skin can thicken and take on a leathery, dry, dull appearance. Daily brushing is an ancient secret for retaining a vibrant, soft, glowing complexion.

The skin is the largest organ of elimination, known as the third kidney in holistic health. It is said that if the internal organs of elimination cannot keep up with the elimination of waste material, then the skin will take over the task. Skin brushing is a valuable addition to your morning routine and can be followed with a cool shower or Epsom salt bath. The invigorating brushing is invaluable to remove dead skin cells, allowing your skin to breathe while creating super soft skin. More importantly, regular skin brushing will support detoxification and waste removal via the lymphatic system.

### Benefits of Dry Skin Brushing
1. **Jump start the lymphatic system**: Skin brushing assists the process of cleansing and detoxification by encouraging lymphatic drainage, speeding up removal of waste matter through the lymph vessels, improving venous circulation while encouraging the elimination of metabolic waste from our tissues. Unlike the heart ,which is an automatic pumping machine, the lymphatic system relies upon the movement of surrounding muscles to keep fluid flowing and effective. Lymphatic congestion can contribute to swelling, fluid retention, inflammation, and chronic disease. In conditions of bed rest, chronic illness, or a sedentary lifestyle, the lymph can become congested and not drain as effectively. This is why movement is essential for our health.
2. Skin brushing **stimulates circulation** by getting the blood flow moving to the extremities, increasing blood flow through the veins and back to the heart while eliminating metabolic waste and cellular debris.

3.  Ensures **normal secretion of sweat and oil glands** for the appearance of moisture-filled, soft and supple skin. In addition, gentle friction over the body's connective tissues and joints will help increase the production of collagen and elastin fibers, going a long way to slow the body's aging process.
4.  **Can improve digestion, assist with regular bowel function, and support the health of the kidneys** through the repetitive and gentle stimulation of the underlying organs. Brush over the abdomen in a clockwise motion, mirroring the direction of the digestive tract (starting at the lower right quadrant, moving up to the belly button, and then over and down the left quadrant of the abdomen). Bloating and fluid retention may diminish as *the body sheds excess fluid and toxins.*
5.  **Skin Exfoliation:** Dry skin brushing removes dead cells, leaving skin super soft and allowing your skin to "breathe."
6.  **Can support breakdown of cellulite**, remove agents which break down connective tissue, improve muscle tone, promote better distribution of fatty deposits, help remove congestion from local veins, and improve lymphatic stagnation.

## Functions of the Lymphatic System

If you are not moving, chances are that your lymph is not moving either! The lymphatic system is dependent upon body movement to move waste material out of the body! Lymphatic vessels:

- Drain waste products from the tissues to your blood for elimination, a process referred to as lymphatic drainage.
- Collects fat and fat-soluble nutrients from intestines.
- Drains fluid from bodily tissues back to the heart.
- Traps debris (toxins, infectious agents) and sends for removal.
- Exercise, stretching, yoga, dry skin brushing, lymphatic drainage massage, hydrotherapy showers, vibration machines, rebounders and lymphatic herbs are all supportive for lymphatic health and efficient waste removal.

## Skin Brushing as part of a daily mindfulness ritual

Each morning dry skin brushing is an invigorating way to start the day. Stay present, put your intention on gratitude, and focus on the optimal outcome for your day while invigorating the body; this practice has been said to stimulate the vital "chi" energy.

Brushing at night is a bit like a meditation; take a couple of minutes to brush down the skin before a nightly Epsom salt bath to unwind, release tension, and relax muscles.

For those who do not take regular massage, or for those who are less active, brushing is effective support for vibrant soft skin and to support the lymphatic system in doing its job.

Skin brushing is done on dry skin by using a dry bristle brush prior to showering or relaxing in a bath. Purchase a natural bristle brush (made from vegetable fibers—do not use a brush made from synthetic fibers or animal bristles). The brush will feel hard and a bit shocking for a new brusher. Persevere—your skin will thank you! Softer brushes can be used on the face. Periodically the bristle brush can be cleaned by using a mild cleanser or castile soap and left to air dry.

## How to Dry Brush Your Skin

Begin with the extremities first: starting from the arms and feet, brush in short circular motions and work towards the heart. Moving from the legs up to the abdomen, brush the abdomen in a clockwise manner, the buttocks and back, the fingers up the arms, and move in the direction of the heart. Avoid brushing areas of thin skin such as the breasts and neck and avoid open wounds, varicose veins, and areas of infection. Do not skin brush during cancer treatment if the tumor has metastasized.

*A body at rest stays at rest. A body in motion stays in motion. No matter what state of health you are in, movement is your friend.*

## Castor Oil Packs

Castor oil is extracted from the seeds of the tropical Castor plant (*Ricinus communis*). One of its common names, palm of Christ, or Palma Christi, was given from the plant's reputed ability to heal wounds. The seeds are rich in triglycerides, mainly ricinolein, an unsaturated omega-9 fatty acid, found to have pain-relieving and anti-inflammatory effects in the body. Ricinolein is thought to increase T-cell receptor signaling (influencing general immunity) and reduce inflammation.

Although internal ingestion of castor oil has been employed tradition-ally as a strong cathartic, moving the bowels in a dynamic way, relieving constipation, and sometimes being used to start an overdue labor, I do not recommend it for internal use; it is simply too strong. That said, when applied externally to the body, castor oil has powerful healing properties. The anti-inflammatory oil is warming to the tissues, thus aids in reducing muscle stiffness, congestion, and pain. Castor oil, when heated, pene-trates through the skin and muscles, affects the underlying tissues, and encourages the breakdown of inflammatory material through enhancing both blood circulation and lymphatic flow. Castor oil increases elimination, improves circulation, and stimulates the activity and movement of lym-phatic fluid (assisting cell detoxification and the excretion of waste mate-rial). Traditional uses include a topical antiseptic application for ringworm, liver spots and warts, athlete's foot, even styes (an infection of the oil glands on the eyelid). Castor oil packs are often applied on the right hand side of the abdomen above the liver, over the whole abdomen or the lower abdomen in the case of reproductive issues, cramping, or pelvic congestion, and over areas of pain, inflammation, or sore muscles. Like all new applica-tions, first test on a small amount of the skin before applying to the whole abdomen or body part.

## Apply a Castor Oil Pack for . . .

- Constipation and sluggish digestion

- Pelvic congestion

- Abdominal swellings and inflammation

- Arthritis and rheumatism

- Muscle spasms and cramping

- Lymphatic congestion

- Fibromyalgia

- Joint stiffness, muscle tension

- Adhesions and scar tissue

- Uterine Cysts, Fibroids, Endometriosis

- Backache

- Hemorrhoids and skin lesions

## How to Apply a Castor Oil Pack

Castor oil packs require commitment, but if used regularly for chronic conditions, it will pay off. The packs should be kept in place for 45 minutes to 1 hour (or many people keep the pack on overnight—with protective bed coverings!). Take a tea towel or flannel cloth large enough to cover the localized area and fold 2–3 times thick. Pour castor oil into a pan and just heat the oil until it is as warm as can be tolerated on the skin (test on your wrist). Soak the cloth in the oil until thoroughly saturated, then squeeze off any excess and place the cloth over the area requiring treatment. Cover with saran wrap or a plastic covering. Then place a heating pad or hot rice pack on top. Many people use this time for relaxation, positive reflection, reading, or meditation. Keep the pack as hot as can be tolerated without burning the skin (reheating the rice pack when necessary) and leave in place for a minimum of 45 minutes or longer. Consider sleeping with this pack on overnight and removing in the morning. To remove the oily film from the skin, use a castile soap mixed with baking soda and wash with warm water. When the application is completed, wrap the cloth in plastic and store in the fridge until ready to reuse. Simply heat more castor oil in a pan and resoak the flannel before reapplying.

Avoid heat applications for situations of active infections, bleeding conditions, or immediate injury. Heat the castor oil on the stove rather than using the microwave. Consistency will pay off; repeat for consecutive days for chronic, long-term ailments. Try using the packs 4 days in a row. Then take a break for 2 days and resume until benefit is noted.

### Ensuring Beautiful Bodies—Inside and Out!

The jury is in: what we put on our skin is absorbed into our bodies and has a long-lasting impact on our health. Society has come a long way from the historical practices of women using arsenic on their skin for a creamy white complexion (in the short term). Remember Queen Elizabeth I and her laborious morning routine consisting of arsenic and lead-containing skin whiteners? However, many chemical ingredients found in cosmetic products today are not much cleaner. A woman may absorb up to five pounds of toxic chemicals through the skin each year.[253]

**Why Create Your Body Care Products At Home?**

- You have 100 % control over what you are putting on and in your body.
- Minimize allergic reactions and chemical sensitivities that cause local inflammation, rashes, and dermatitis.
- Eliminate toxic chemicals in commercial products, known as endocrine disruptors, hormone imbalancers, xenoestrogens and carcinogens as well as their cumulative effects on hormonal, reproductive and thyroid functions, obesity, immune regulation, and development of various cancers.
- Environmental consideration—xenoestrogens not only have an impact on our health but impact marine life and small animals. Once these chemicals get into our water supply, nothing is immune.
- They are cost-effective, often costing a fraction of brand name items.
- An opportunity to teach our children and future generations about the impact consumer choices have on our long-term health and the health of the environment.

## EXFOLIANTS AND SCRUBS

Instead of using plastic beads, natural face and body scrubs can act as skin exfoliators using oatmeal, poppy seeds, coffee, or almond meal, effectively removing dead skin cells and creating a healthy glow. If the end goal is to remove dead cells while allowing our skin to breathe, then we don't want to be coating our skin with problematic chemicals. In my experience, body care blends made at home work far more effectively than a commercial or brand name product. Give them a try! Exfoliants should be avoided over areas of open wounds, infection, or irritated skin.

# Body Scrub Exfoliant

## Ingredients
2 cups Epsom Salt
¼ cup Coconut Oil
2 tablespoons Grape-seed Oil
3 drops Lavender Essential Oil

## Directions
In a medium bowl, combine Epsom salts, oil, and essential oil. Mix well. Prior to a bath, rub the salt mixture into just moistened skin, working gently into rough areas or dry patches of skin. Then enjoy a bathtub soak! The end result is soft, glowing skin and improved circulation.

# Start the Day Right Stimulating Coffee Scrub

**Ingredients**
4 parts organic Coffee grounds
1 part Olive Oil or salt
Warm Water—just enough to moisten the mixture and apply to the skin

**Directions**
Combine coffee grounds with water and olive oil or salt. The choice is yours. Olive oil is moisturizing for dry skin while the salt is more drying and pulling for impurities and oily skin. Or simply use fresh water with coffee grounds. Mix in enough warm water to mix well. Rub into the body while in the shower. Place a fine mesh in the drain to prevent clogging. For those who prefer coffee first: before a shower, scoop out some of the wet grounds from your morning coffee and use as a morning scrub.

# All Over Soothing Oatmeal Scrub

Oatmeal is an emollient for face and body recipes; it softens the skin, removes dirt, and provides soothing properties for dry skin, acne, and rashes, as well as anti-itch effects for poison ivy, dermatitis, and sunburn.

**Ingredients**
½ cup Oatmeal
3 tablespoons dried Rose petals
3 tablespoons Lavender flowers
Coffee Grinder

**Directions**
Place ingredients in the coffee grinder and grind until finely powdered. Store in a glass container. When ready to apply, mix with 1 teaspoon of water or some olive oil (for a hydrating blend). Very gently rub into your skin in circular motions. Let sit for a couple of minutes, then rinse.

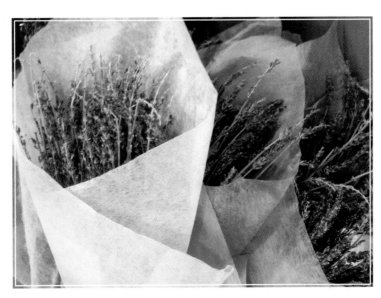

# You're So Sweet Facial Scrub

There was a time when my home was absent of sugar in all forms; when ingested, sugar is a poison for the body. Thus I feel that its best use is ON the body, not in it!

## Ingredients
½ teaspoon Honey
1 teaspoon raw organic Cane sugar
1 teaspoon fresh Lemon juice

## Directions
Combine sugar with the honey, squeeze in the lemon juice, mix well, and apply to the face in circular motions. If the mix is too runny, simply add more sugar. Prepare a larger volume to store in a container for daily use.

# BAKING SODA FACIAL SCRUB

For removal of whiteheads, blackheads, enlarged pores, and for acne-prone skin, give this simple blend a try.

**Ingredients**
Baking Soda
Water

**Directions**
Make a paste with water and baking soda. Apply onto moistened skin and work into the skin for a couple of minutes in a circular motion. Leave on 2–3 minutes before washing off. *Optional: the baking soda can be mixed into your favorite cleanser or 1 teaspoon of the juice of a fresh lemon can be used for oily skin.

## The Bounty of Baking Soda

Back in the late 1700s, baking soda was created from sodium carbonate. As I recall from childhood, the baking soda found its home in the fridge as a reliable air freshener. There are numerous applications for baking soda. It is a reliable cleaning agent—used with vinegar and lemons, it can be used on pots and pans to remove burnt blackened bits or as a base for toothpaste. When mixed with water it can be used weekly as a skin exfoliant to remove impurities and cleanse pores for a clear complexion.

| Baking Soda Benefits—The Wonders of Sodium Bicarbonate |
| --- |
| Disinfectant and antifungal properties |
| Antacid, heartburn support: when mixed with water, use only in moderation |
| Home Cleaning agent: cutting grease, air freshener |
| Fire extinguisher for shallow pans: Baking soda releases carbon dioxide when heated, keeping oxygen out of the fire and smothering the flame. Don't use in oil fires from deep pans to avoid splattering the oil |
| Pest control: sprinkle in corners where cockroaches linger |
| Anti-itch remedy: hives, poison ivy, allergic reactions |
| Topical powder mixed with water for pulling out splinters from the skin |
| Body care ingredient: bath salts, toothpaste, exfoliants, mouthwash |

# Avocado, Rose, and Carrot Skin Mask

Apply to dry, aging, delicate skin—nourishing for the face, elbows, and calloused feet.

**Ingredients**
1 Carrot, medium size
½ Avocado
1 tablespoon Olive Oil
5 drops Avocado Oil
1 drop Rose Essential Oil
1 tablespoon Epsom Salt (for sensitive skin, use ½ teaspoon of Baking Soda instead)

**Directions**
Steam carrot until soft and mash in a bowl. Cut half an avocado, scoop out the meat, add into the bowl plus olive oil, avocado oil, rose essential oil, and Epsom salt or soda. Mix well. Apply the mixture to damp, freshly-bathed skin. Rub in a circular motion to gently exfoliate the dead skin from the area. Let sit for 15 minutes. Wash with warm water.

# Nourishing Avocado Facial Mask

**Ingredients**
½ Avocado
2 tablespoon Honey
1 tablespoon natural cold Yogurt or 1 teaspoon Coconut Oil

**Directions**
Remove the pit from half an avocado and slice the avocado into squares
for easy blending; lift the flesh out of the peel and into a bowl. With a fork,
mash the avocado until creamy and free from lumps. Mix in all ingredients.
Apply to the face uniformly, avoiding the eyes. Let sit and dry. Reapply
more than one layer on the skin. Rinse with warm water. Leave on your face
for about 20 minutes. Enjoy immediate, soothing relief for tight, dry, aging
skin; also ideal for large pores to astringe, tighten, and cleanse pores.

# Papaya, Honey, and Jojoba Oily Skin Mask

**Ingredients**
$1/3$ cup ripe Papaya, peeled, seeded, and pureed
3 teaspoons of Oatmeal, powdered
¼ cup Honey
1 teaspoon Jojoba oil
4 drops Rose Geranium Essential Oil

**Directions**
Blend together and apply to acne-prone skin. After 10 minutes, wash off
with warm water. This antiaging mask helps reduce skin inflammation,
draws out impurities, and helps minimize excess oil.

# PINEAPPLE MINT SKIN TONER

## Ingredients
1 teaspoon Spearmint herb (dried or 3 teaspoons fresh)
1 teaspoon Pineapple weed (dried or 3 teaspoons fresh)
2 cups distilled Water
1 teaspoon Witch Hazel Water

## Directions
Prepare an infusion by steeping herbs for 15 minutes, then strain. Poor the
cooled tea into a spritzer bottle and use on the skin for an invigorating,
soothing astringent for tightening pores. Lasts for 2 weeks or keep cold
for a longer shelf life. Use to remove makeup, tighten pores, and soothe
inflamed skin.

# Yarrow and Red Raspberry Astringent

## Ingredients
1 teaspoon Yarrow dried leaf or flower
1 teaspoon Red Raspberry dried herb
½ cup distilled Water
2 teaspoons Witch Hazel Water (alcohol free is best for oily skin)

## Directions
Prepare a strong infusion using equal portions of the herbs in the water, then mix in the witch hazel water following the instructions above—for oily skin.

## Cleanser for Clogged Pores
Are blackheads or congested pores a nagging problem? A simple solution for clogged pores is a back-to-the-basics blend using the astringency of a fresh Lemon, and the pulling power of Salt and Water. Add in a drop of Lavender essential oil as an antiseptic and anti-inflammatory, and see just how clear your skin will become.

# LEMON PORE TREATMENT

Use as a great support for problem skin with enlarged pores.

## Ingredients
2 tablespoons of Sea Salt
1 teaspoon of freshly-squeezed Lemon juice
1 tablespoon warm Water
1 drop Lavender Essential Oil

## Directions
Mix together and apply to a moistened face. Work the mixture into the skin in circular motions using your fingers; keep reapplying the mixture. In my experience, the localized skin will become a bit red during this stage, but calms down minutes later. Apply a warm, moist facecloth to the face and rub in a circular motion. Wash off with cold water. After the application, my own skin is smooth and clear, and the pores are noticeably smaller, tighter, and less congested. Reapply a couple times a week, as needed, to keep the pores clear. This recipe can be doubled for application on the neck, back, chest, or any problem areas containing blackheads and clogged pores.

## BATHS AND SOAKS
### Epsom Salt Baths
Epsom salts are named from a natural salt spring near Epsom in England. The natural salts are composed from magnesium sulfate (magnesium, sulfur, and oxygen together) with water molecules attached. Magnesium is an essential nutrient used to regulate many enzymes in the body, from decreasing inflammation to supporting nerve function. Epsom salt (magnesium sulphate) baths are a traditional remedy used to relax tight muscles, promote a restful sleep, improve circulation, support lymphatic and liver congestion, treat colds and flus, to assist arthritis, treat athletic injuries and stiff muscles as well as helping all conditions of toxemia. It is also a great way to relax the muscles and calm the mind to prepare for a rest-filled sleep. There are many foot problems that can be treated with Epsom salts.

Joint pain, swollen feet, toe fungus, and foot odor can all be improved by soaking in a warm Epsom salt footbath. Soaking the whole body or the affected body part in a hot solution will encourage fresh blood supply to the area, providing healing nutrients and oxygen while at the same time encouraging the release of accumulated toxins that predispose one to irritation and inflammation.

**Think of Epsom Salts for:**
- Sore, tight muscles and joint pain
- Promoting sleep, encouraging relaxation
- Rheumatism, gout pain, arthritis
- Detoxification, sweating out toxins through the skin
- Skin exfoliation
- Insect bites
- Poison Ivy
- Swollen feet
- Toe fungus
- The onset of a cold or flu, to jumpstart the immune system
- Foot soak to relieve odor—steep with sage
- Warming body temperature, improving circulation, warming cold hands and feet

## Muscle Relaxation and Sleep Promotion Epsom Salt Bath
Use 3–4 cups of Epsom salts in a hot bath.
Add 5 drops of Lavender or 2 drops of Chamomile essential oil.
Ease your body into the bath and soak for 10–15 minutes, then head straight to bed for a relaxing sleep. The Epsom salts are relaxing for muscle tension, cramping, and symptoms of joint pain; they are also sleep promoting. An ideal way to end a long day.

## Preparation for Sleep
One of my favorite ways to relax is with candles and a hot bath, with Epsom salts mixed in. Soaking in an Epsom salt bath can help you feel rejuvenated. It will also keep your skin hydrated and healthy and your muscles relaxed.

# BODILICIOUS BATH CRYSTALS

These bath salts are a hit! They are lots of fun to make, inexpensive, and with some creative bottles and labels, make lovely gifts.

## Ingredients
2 cups Epsom Salts
½ cup Pink Himalayan Salt
10 drops Lavender Essential Oil
5 drops Rose Essential Oil
4 tablespoons dried Lavender flowers
4 tablespoons dried Rose flowers
1 tablespoon Marigold flowers
* Fresh flower petals can also be used directly in the bath.

## Directions
Mix the salts, essential oils, and dried flowers together in a medium-sized bowl. Transfer mixture to a small storage jar. Pour these fragrant bath crystals into your bath as desired. Place a strainer in the drain to catch the flower bits before they make their way down the drain. Or fill into a cotton bag or muslin sachet and secure closed for an easier clean.

# Rose Honey Body Moisturizer

**Ingredients**
4 tablespoons Rose petals, dried
2 cups Almond Oil in a medium-size bottle.
5 tablespoons Honey
3 drops Rose Essential Oil
3 drops Vitamin E Oil

**Directions**
Prepare an infused oil of Rose, using 4 tablespoons dried rose petals and 2 cups Almond oil (and following directions on page 233). Heat for 3 hours at a low temperature in double boiler or Crock-pot; do not burn the oil. Remove from heat, strain, cool, and mix in honey, vitamin E, and essential oil. Bottle. Apply to the body as a moisturizer.

# Basil Lavender Natural Deodorant

## Ingredients
2 teaspoons Coconut Oil
8 drops Rose Geranium Essential Oil
8 drops Basil Essential Oil
8 drops Lavender Essential Oil
2 tablespoons Cocoa butter
2 tablespoons Shea butter
½ teaspoon grated Beeswax for a more solid consistency
2 tablespoons Arrowroot powder
1 tablespoon Baking Soda
5 drops Vitamin E Oil

## Directions
In a double boiler, combine the oils, butters, and beeswax together; gently heat until melted. Remove from heat and stir in arrowroot powder, baking soda, vitamin E, adding in your essential oil blend last. Pour into jars. Cover with a paper towel and let sit until cool and solid—about 5 hours or overnight. Place the lids on securely and apply a small amount as needed in the morning to the underarms and on your feet as well, if needed. Options: Grapefruit and Basil, Orange and Lavender essential oils are other possible scents. Or choose your own favorite blend.

## FOR THE FEET
Herbal infusions and essential oils can go a long way to restoring aching, swollen feet. Epsom salt baths, peppermint and spearmint, self-heal, and marigold can all invigorate our feet, providing antifungal properties.

When travelling, I frequently prepare footbaths after a long day of walking to rejuvenate and refresh tired feet. A couple drops of lavender or peppermint essential oil works wonders for tired feet.

# Marigold Nail Fungus Soak

**Ingredients**
3 tablespoons Marigold flowers
2 cups Water
1 cup Apple Cider Vinegar
4 tablespoons of Baking Soda

**Directions**
Brew the marigold flowers as an infusion with boiling water in a bowl. Steep 15 minutes. Add in one cup of vinegar and 4 tablespoons of baking soda. Soak the area of fungus for 10 minutes. Repeat twice a day.

Other herbs that can be used topically include: oregano, thyme, goldenrod, rosemary, and self-heal.

**Summer Plantar Warts**

Summer weather means walking barefoot, afternoons at the local pool, and an increased risk of plantar warts, which are caused by the human papillomavirus, a virus that thrives in warm, moist environments. Here are some natural options to try.

| Traditional Wart Applications |
| --- |
| Garlic juice applied twice daily and crushed garlic applied at night—secure with band aid |
| Unpasteurized Honey applied in a bandage—apply to wart |
| Dandelion Stem Milk applied directly to wart frequently |
| Peel of a ripe Banana secure to wart nightly |
| Tea Tree Essential Oil, Cinnamon Essential Oil, Lemon Essential Oil topically on wart |
| Apple Cider Vinegar—soaked in cotton and secured over the wart. Apply twice daily |
| Raw onion and salt applied morning and night |

**Insect Bite First Aid**

Obtain medical attention immediately if experiencing breathing difficulties, wheezing, swelling of the tongue, face, or lips, or if the area around the bite becomes discolored.

For tick removal: Remove tick with fine tipped tweezers by pulling the tick straight out of the body. Save the tick in a jar to test in case one experiences flu-like symptoms and a red rash after the bite.

# PLANT MINT BITE BALM

## Ingredients
2 cups boiling hot Water
2 tablespoons Plantain leaf
2 tablespoons Epsom Salts
1–2 drops Peppermint Essential Oil

## Directions
Boil water. Place the water in a bowl and add in plantain. First brew as a tea, covered for 10 minutes. Strain. Stir in the Epsom salts and dissolve. Add a drop of peppermint essential oil. Soak a facecloth and apply to insect bites for immediate anti-inflammatory relief. Or if you are out in a field, simply find plantain and implement the spit poultice!

# POISON IVY RELIEF

## Ingredients
2 cups Epsom Salts
1 cup Baking Soda
Cool water in a bath
5 drops Lavender Essential Oil
3 drops Peppermint Essential Oil
Cotton washcloth

## Directions
Add all ingredients to the tub. Dissolve the crystals in the bath, then ease your way in. Add ice cubes to cool down the water. Soak the cotton washcloth and apply to the affected area as needed. This application can also be prepared in a basin for more localized areas. Add in ice cubes for cooling relief. Apply a paste of baking soda powder (moistened with a little water to form a paste) to the rash after the bath. The baking soda and peppermint essential oil will be a welcome relief from the itchiness.

### Anti-Itch Oatmeal Paste
Just like preparing breakfast, cook a small amount of oatmeal on the stove. Cool slightly prior to applying to the skin, to ensure you do not burn (test by putting a small amount on your wrist), and apply it directly to the skin as a paste. Add just enough water so the oatmeal is thick and will cling or hold to the skin. Apply and wait until the oatmeal is completely cool. Rinse the skin. Baking soda and 1–2 drops of peppermint essential oil can be added for an extra itch-relieving effect. Soothing relief from poison ivy, itchy skin rashes, and dermatitis.

| Rash Relief: Poison Ivy, Hives, Itching Skin |
| --- |
| Oatmeal baths, poultices, ground powder mixed with water |
| Organic Alcohol-free Witch Hazel Water—cooling and astringent to tissues |
| Aloe Vera—Use the inner gel of the plant or purchase commercial pure aloe gel—should only contain one preservative! Read your labels. |
| Cucumber puree or slices will help to cool itching skin |
| Chickweed<br>Plantain |
| Alterative Plants internally as a tea: Nettles, Red Clover, Dandelion, Cleavers Baking soda paste, salt, yogurt—all provide cooling effects |

### Burn Relief

**Lavender flowers or Marigold flowers:** prepare an infusion. Prepare as a tea and soak cotton in the tea (follow the poultice or fomentation directions); apply to the affected areas, leaving on 20–30 minutes.

**Lavender essential oil:** applied directly to the skin, for relief of sunstroke, burns, fainting, and boils.

**Peppermint essential oil:** mixes well with Aloe vera gel as cooling relief for burns.

**Aloe vera juice:** excellent healing plant to keep in your home. Apply the leaves directly to the affected areas. (If using bottled Aloe, look for the one that is 98% pure, without a long list of colorings and preservatives, and keep refrigerated once opened.) See page 124 for application of Lavender essential oil on burns.

# Soothe Away the Ouch Sunburn Blend

## Ingredients
50 ml Aloe Vera Juice or Gel
20 ml Witch Hazel, distilled
10 drops of Lavender Essential Oil
3 drops Peppermint Essential Oil
20 ml Spearmint herb infusion
10 ml distilled Water

## Directions
Mix together all ingredients in a spray bottle. Shake well. Apply liberally and frequently to cool a burn.

### For Cuts
Cayenne pepper is a hemostatic herb! What does it do? It stops bleeding! I keep this powder handy in the first aid cabinet for any open cut or wound. Sprinkle the powder over a bleeding wound and watch the blood clot in front of your eyes.

## Coconut Oil

Coconut oil is an herbalist's joy, offering a variety of options for skin and body care. It becomes liquid around 24 degrees Celsius, however it is solid at cooler temperatures and can be used in cooking oil, for dry hair, as a moisturizer (it is one of the very best natural lubricants) and it's edible (with no preservatives!). Coconut oil contains Caprylic and Lauric acids, which provide natural antifungal and antibacterial properties beneficial to the shelf life of a product and to deter candida. Coconut oil is a medium chained triglyceride; when consumed, it is metabolized by the liver in a way that provides immediate energy and ketones that support mental health and enhance cognitive function.

I choose certified organic, virgin, cold-pressed, unrefined coconut oil which is bottled in a glass container. The coconut oil retains the delicious coconut scent. Also I look for products labelled hexane free, as many companies can use toxic solvents in the manufacturing process and I support monkey-friendly companies! As consumers select healthier choices at home, it is essential that the shift supports the larger goal—sustainable practices for the health of the environment—and guarantee that no animals are harmed or abused for the latest human trend. Monkey labor is common in the commercial harvesting of ripe coconuts; monkeys can be forced to harvest up to one thousand coconuts per day. With no opportunity to socialize as monkeys, they have been trained to serve the interests and free labor of man. It is worth the couple extra dollars to support fair-trade, sustainable practices for the livelihood of everyone on this planet, especially animals. Support companies that support sustainable, clean products and consciously take steps not to harm animals for our commercial needs.

# Herbal Hair Rinse

## Ingredients
1 teaspoon dried Nettle leaf
1 teaspoon dried Rosemary leaf
1 teaspoon dried Sage leaf
Hot water
½ cup Apple Cider Vinegar

## Directions
Prepare an infusion using 1 teaspoon of each of the herbs to 2 cups water; steep 15 minutes. Strain and add in the ½ cup apple cider vinegar. Use weekly as a hair rinse, after shampooing to remove buildup of hair products, stimulate scalp circulation, and promote hair growth.

**Traditional Honey Hair Conditioner**
Use as a traditional blend for hydrating the hair. Mix equal portions of honey and olive oil. Cover hair with a shower cap and sit for 30 minutes. Shampoo out.

## Topical Treatments

The health of the hair and the skin is an indication of the health of the internal body.

As a teenager perusing teen magazines for beauty tips, I had my share of sleepovers that unfolded into a beauty spa event with face masks and hair masks. Avocados, eggs, honey, and yogurt were the key ingredients for face masks and body care blends. We tried them all—the prepackaged body care products with a long list of chemical names that I still cannot pronounce and the natural recipes involving gobs of egg and chunks of avocado everywhere. Although messy for a group of girls at a sleepover, they were effective. We all had long hair and the avocado mask was one of my favorites for moisturizing curly dry hair. Years later, natural recipes are still my preference for healthy hair and deep-conditioning treatments.

The same nourishing fats and oils in avocado that contribute to deep hydration for your body are also a great option to help tame and repair dry, frizzy, brittle, or damaged hair. Chemically colored hair will respond to this treatment as well. Olive oil is extremely hydrating, and when my naturally curly hair is just a little too out of control and I am too busy to prepare a full hair treatment, I simply slather olive oil into my hair and ends before bed and wash out in the morning.

# HONEY YOUR HAIR LOOKS LOVELY FORMULA FOR DRY FRIZZY HAIR

## Ingredients
1 ripe Avocado or 3 tablespoons Avocado Oil
3 tablespoons Olive Oil
4 tablespoons Honey
2–3 drops Rosemary or Lavender Essential Oil

## Directions
In a small mixing bowl, mash an avocado, adding olive oil, honey, and essential oils. Blend until smooth. Dampen hair or apply after a shower. Work well into the hair, rubbing it into the scalp and the ends, which are generally drier. Twist up hair and clip to top of head. Cover with a shower cap and heat. Warm with a hair dryer or use the sun's rays. Leave on 15–30 minutes. Remove shower cap, rinse mask, and then wash hair as usual.

# Banana and Carrot Deep Hair Conditioner

In need of a deep conditioner to bring back the shine to dull lifeless hair?

**Ingredients**
1 ripe Banana
1 Carrot (steam soft or use carrot juice)
2 tablespoons creamy Yogurt
½ Avocado
1 teaspoon of Coconut Oil
1 teaspoon Honey

**Directions**
Cut the banana into a bowl. Steam the carrot until soft, then mash with the banana. Add yogurt, avocado, coconut oil, and honey. Blend together until smooth. Apply to the full length of the hair and massage into the scalp. Cover hair with a shower cap and leave on for 30 minutes to an hour. Apply heat to encourage a deeper conditioning. Use a hair dryer or sit outside under the sun. Rinse hair and shampoo. Style as usual.

# STRAWBERRY HAIR MASK

Need a use for overripe Strawberries? Consider adding them into a nourishing hair mask.

**Ingredients**
1 cup Strawberries
1 Egg yolk
2 tablespoons Coconut Oil

**Directions**
Puree ingredients in a food processor or hand-held blender and apply to hair.

# CASTOR OIL TREATMENT FOR THINNING HAIR

## Ingredients
3 tablespoons of Castor oil
1 tablespoon Coconut Oil
3 drops of Rosemary Essential Oil

## Directions
Blend ingredients in a jar and shake well. If the coconut oil is solid at room temperature, put the closed container briefly in a bowl of warm water and it will soften soon enough. Apply to the parted sections of the scalp, massaging in circular motions until the entire scalp has been coated. This is a deep conditioning treatment that stimulates circulation for thinning hair, ideal for dry, chemically-treated hair and a dry, flaking scalp. The rosemary essential oil assists with improving circulation to the scalp.

# Herbal Toothpaste

## Ingredients
¼ teaspoon Salt ground into a powder
½ teaspoon Myrrh powder
$1/3$ cup Bentonite clay powder
1 teaspoon Xylitol powder
Approx. 60 ml Spearmint infused tea (prepared from distilled Water)
½ teaspoon Coconut Oil
2 teaspoon Plantain Tincture
1–2 drops Sweet Orange, Clove, or Lemon Essential Oils
¼ teaspoon Baking Soda

## Directions
Mix together the salt, myrrh powder, and clay, using a mortar and pestle to finely powder the ingredients. Add xylitol powder as a sweetener, slightly more or less depending on your taste preference. Mix together and bottle. This dried powder can be shaken onto a toothbrush and used as a tooth powder.

To create a creamy toothpaste, with a shorter shelf life, add in the spearmint tea to form the desired consistency, and add coconut oil, plantain tincture, and essential oils—just 1 or 2 drops of essential oils are needed for flavoring.

The plantain offers pulling powers for infection and gum inflammation. The myrrh and essential oils are antiseptic. Clay contains pulling power, and the baking soda and salt are abrasive.

# HERBAL MOUTH WASH

## Ingredients
1 teaspoon dried Basil leaf
2 tablespoons dried Sage leaf
2 tablespoons dried Plantain leaf
1 tablespoon Rosemary leaf
4 tablespoons boiling Water
250 ml/ 8 ounces Vodka
5 drops of Clove, Orange, or Spearmint Essential Oil
1 teaspoon Vegetable glycerine (optional for flavor)

## Directions
Place the herbs in a wide-mouth glass jar. Pour 4 tablespoons of boiling water over herbs. Cool to room temperature and add vodka into the jar with the herbs. Cover tightly and let sit for 2 weeks, shaking daily to encourage the release of chemical constituents into the menstruum. After 2 weeks, strain the mixture with cheesecloth or a strainer. Discard the herbs, and pour the tincture into a glass bottle. Add the essential oils and glycerine. Shake well before use. Dilute 1 tablespoon into 2 ounces of warm water and use as a mouthwash.

# LAVENDER HOPS EYE PILLOWS

## Ingredients
½ cup dried Lavender flowers
1 tablespoon dried Hops strobiles
½ cup Flaxseeds
2 drops Lavender Essential Oil
Two 7 x 3.5-inch rectangles of Silk fabric

## Directions
Obtain colorful soft silk fabric and cut into two 7 x 3.5-inch rectangles.
Place both sides of the fabric inside out. Stitch 3 sides closed (by hand or
with a sewing machine) leaving one of the 3.5-inch sides open for filling.
Then turn the fabric right side out. Mix the lavender, Hops, and flaxseeds
together and drop in the essential oil. Fill into the pillow. The pillow should
be bendable and not completely packed. Stitch closed. Use at nighttime.
Place the pillow over closed eyes; the weight will help to relax the eye
muscles (for eye strain) and provide a soothing sedative effect to welcome
dream time.

# For the Home

**INSECT REPELLENTS**

In an open window, hang cotton ribbons with a few drops of essential oil added. Choose to grow herbs in the garden with insect-repellent properties. Consider the daisy and pineapple weed insect repellant from page 127. Infusions of herbs can be brewed and mixed into a spritzer bottle, diluted in water for spritzing on the skin.

For topical relief of heat and swelling of insect bites, apply a poultice, wash, or cream containing turmeric, chickweed, heartsease, feverfew, self-heal, plantain, and watercress.

### Essential Oil Insect Repellents

- Flies and moths: Lavender essential oil
- Fleas: Lavender, Citronella, Eucalyptus
- Mosquitoes: Peppermint essential oil
- Ants: Peppermint, Citronella
- Lice: Tea Tree, Cinnamon and Thyme essential oils mixed in Apple Cider Vinegar

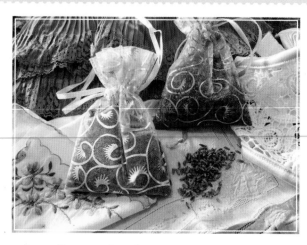

# Lavender Spearmint Moth Repellent Sachets

**Ingredients**
$1/3$ cup dried Spearmint leaf
$1/3$ cup dried Lavender flowers
3 drops Lavender Essential Oil

**Directions**
Mix together in a bowl and fill a cotton sachet. Place between sheets and blankets in the linen closet, layer between wool sweaters to protect from moths, or hang from a coat hanger. Used to help keep fabric smelling fresh and offer insect-repellent properties for moths, silverfish, and ants. Refresh the Lavender essential oil periodically and crush the flowers to release more volatile oils.

## ENVIRONMENTALLY FRIENDLY HOME CLEANSERS
Household cleaning agents hold health concerns due to toxic ingredients. Have you ever observed the skull and crossbones warning on the containers and wondered: what is in these cleansers and why are there no ingredients listed on the outside of the bottle?

If you have young children who play on the carpet or naturally curious four-legged friends that are notorious for walking on freshly washed floors, take note: if the floor was cleaned with toxic agents, residues on tiny paws or small fingers can be ingested. Consider stocking up on some basic items to create natural cleaning products, and create your own cleaning agents.

**Basic Ingredients:** Vinegar, Baking Soda, Fresh Lemons, and Essential Oils

**All-Purpose Cleaner:** Mix 5 tablespoons baking soda with 1 quart warm water. Add 10 drops of Lemon, Grapefruit, or Orange essential oil.

**Carpet Cleaner:** Lightly sprinkle baking soda over the carpet and rub it in. After 1 hour, drop 5–6 drops of Lemon or Orange essential oil on the carpet and then vacuum up the soda. For tough stains, use cold baking soda water or blot the area with vinegar and soapy water.

**Counter Stains:** Apply fresh lemon juice, then scrub with baking soda and watch stains disappear.

**Deodorizer:** Keep a spray bottle filled with pure (5 percent acetic acid) white vinegar for cleaning near the cutting board. Just spray it on, let sit, and wipe off. Option: Add in Lemon, Orange, or Tea Tree essential oil for a light, clean scent and added antiseptic properties.

**Disinfectant:** Mix 2 tablespoons of vinegar, 10 drops of Lemon and Orange essential oil, 3 drops of Cinnamon, and ¼ cup of castile soap with 2 cups of hot water or 3 percent hydrogen peroxide poured in a spritzer bottle: use to wipe down doorknobs, home telephone handset, countertops, children's toys, boxes . . . basically anything requiring disinfecting!

**Drain Cleaner:** Pour ¼ cup of salt and ¼ cup of baking soda down the drain. Add ½ cup of vinegar. Wait 15 minutes, and then flush the drain with boiling water.

**Grease stains:** For clothing, rub on moistened baking soda to treat the stain, and launder.

**Fridge Cleaner:** Wipe down shelves with 2 cups of hot water, ½ cup white vinegar, and ¼ cup hydrogen peroxide. Then rinse with castile soap in hot water.

**Wood Furniture Polish:** Mix ¼ cup of vinegar or use ¼ cup fresh lemon juice in ½ cup of vegetable oil and apply with a clean rag to buff up wood surfaces. Place in sealed container and store for future use.

**Glass Cleaner:** Mix ½ cup of white vinegar with 1 gallon of warm water in a spray bottle.

**Stove Cleaner:** Apply a thick paste of baking soda and water, let it sit overnight and then scrub with a cloth.

**Sweat Stains on Clothing:** White vinegar and water (1:4 ratio) to cover the stain. Soak for 12 hours, then wash.

**Oil stains on Clothing:** Pretreat the stain by using baking soda moistened with water, then wash.

**Toilet Bowl Cleaner:** Use baking soda and white vinegar. Sprinkle baking soda into the toilet bowl. Add vinegar. Add 3–4 drops of essential oil for added disinfectant power. Scour with a toilet brush.

**Tile Cleaner:** Use toothbrush, moistened, with baking soda. Dilute 3 parts baking soda mixed with 1 part water. Or alternatively, use 3 percent hydrogen peroxide, spray on the tiles or areas of mildew and let sit before cleaning. Use in the bathroom for the tub and surrounding tile.

**Weed Killer:** Mix ½ gallon apple cider vinegar with 1/3 cup salt and 1 tablespoon dish soap. Kills weeds (and plants) it comes in contact with. Apply selectively.

# Glossary of Herbal Medicine

**Adaptogens:** Herbs that help our bodies adapt to stress (both internal and external stress) by supporting the adrenal glands, immune system function, the endocrine system, and enhancing the stamina and vitality of the whole person.

**Alterative:** Traditionally known as "blood cleansers," these herbs help to improve the health and vitality of the body by supporting the organs and aiding the removal of metabolic toxins. Examples: burdock, cleavers, nettles, red clover, dandelion, marigold, cabbage, parsley, heartsease, cleavers, juniper

**Amphoteric:** A normalizer—an herb that harmonizes and normalizes the function of an organ or body system, balancing two seemingly contradictory conditions such as diarrhea and constipation. Examples: cayenne, lavender, red raspberry

**Analgesic or anodynes:** These herbs reduce or eliminate pain (used internally or topically). Examples: chamomile, lavender, feverfew, California poppy, ginger, cayenne, oregano, juniper, hops

**Anthelmintic:** Herbs that destroy and dispel worms and parasites from the body. (Also known as vermicides or vermifuges).

**Anodyne:** Herbs that relieve pain and reduce sensitivity of the nerves. (See analgesic)

**Antibiotic:** Inhibits the growth of germs, bacteria, and harmful microbes (used either internally or topically). Examples: thyme, rosemary, oregano, onion

**Anticatarrhal**: Herbs that assist in the removal of excess phlegm from the nose, throat, sinuses. Examples: goldenrod, thyme, yarrow, nettle, horseradish, chamomile, marigold, plantain

**Antidiabetic**: Agents that assist in blood sugar management. Examples: fenugreek, cinnamon, dandelion root, nettle, garlic, turmeric, burdock

**Antidiarrheals**: Herbs that astringe and soothe an irritated bowel. Examples: cinnamon, blackberry, red raspberry, ginger, sunflower, self-heal, plantain, sage

**Anti-emetic**: Prevents, helps to reduce, or alleviates nausea and vomiting. Examples: ginger, lemon balm, red raspberry

**Antifungal**: Herbal agents that can destroy fungus, candida, and thrush (for both internal and external use). Examples: marigold, garlic, oregano, thyme, rosemary, sage

**Antihemorrhagic**: powerful astringents able to arrest mild to moderate bleeding. Examples: cayenne, marigold, plantain, red raspberry, nettles, sage

**Antihistamines**: Agents that stop the production of histamine in the body, used in allergic conditions. Examples: garlic, nettles, chamomile, plantain, Californian poppy

**Anti-inflammatory**: Herbals that help to minimize inflammation and support the body's natural healing process. Examples: chamomile, feverfew, turmeric, cabbage, fennel, parsley, onion, avocado, yarrow, corn silk, pineapple weed, marigold, self-heal, sage, red clover, heartsease, sweet violet, cleavers, rosemary, mullein, goldenrod, juniper, rose hips

**Antilithic**: Assist to prevent the formation and removal of stones in the kidneys and bladder. Examples: corn silk, dandelion

**Antimicrobial**: Agents that help the body resist or destroy foreign pathogens (containing antiviral and antibacterial properties) by increasing the body's resistance to infection. Examples: oregano, garlic, thyme, marigold, sage, rosemary, juniper

**Antirheumatic**: Herbs that relieve rheumatism, inflammation, and pain. Examples: feverfew, cayenne, ginger, chickweed, nettles, heartsease, juniper

**Antiscorbutic**: Effective in the prevention or treatment of scurvy.

**Antiseptic**: Prevents decay or putrefaction; a substance that inhibits the growth and development of microorganisms. Examples: thyme, oregano, marigold, sage, rosemary, yarrow, garlic, burdock, sweet violet, mullein, goldenrod

**Antispasmodic**: Relieves or prevents involuntary muscle spasm or smooth muscle cramps. Examples: chamomile, peppermint and spearmint, ginger, feverfew, California poppy, sage, red clover, rosemary, thyme, oregano, juniper, rose hips

**Antitussive**: Prevents or improves a cough. Examples: mullein, thyme, ginger, sunflower, California poppy

**Aromatic**: Herbs containing volatile oils creating a fragrant scent. Examples: aniseed, caraway, chamomile, ginger, spearmint, cinnamon, fennel, turmeric, thyme, rosemary, sage, oregano, juniper, rose, lavender

**Astringent**: Herbs that promote tightening of the tissues, blood vessels, and mucous membranes; used to stop internal bleeding, inflammation , diarrhea, and reduce secretions. Examples: plantain, yarrow, cinnamon, self-heal, cleavers, rosemary, sage, red raspberry, mullein, rose, rose hips

**Bitter**: Taken before a meal, stimulates the appetite, and promotes optimal digestion. Examples: yarrow, marigold, feverfew, dandelion, chamomile, hops, pineapple weed, self-heal, burdock, thyme

**Carminative**: Herbs that helps to prevent cramping, gas and bloating. Examples: chamomile, caraway, aniseed, fennel, spearmint, cinnamon, ginger, horseradish, carrot, onion, turmeric, feverfew, lavender, pineapple weed, sage, rosemary, thyme, oregano, goldenrod, juniper

**Cholagogue**: Plants that stimulate the flow of bile from the liver and gall bladder. Examples: dandelion root, watercress, lavender, marigold, burdock

**Decongestant**: For relieving congestion (see expectorant). Examples: mullein, ginger, horseradish, goldenrod, spearmint

**Demulcent**: An herb that soothes, protects, and relieves the irritation of inflamed mucous membranes. Examples: plantain, corn silk, mullein, borage

**Diaphoretic**: Helps to lower a fever and reduce chills; promotes sweating and increases perspiration by dilating surface capillaries. Examples: yarrow, cayenne, garlic, ginger, cinnamon, chamomile, feverfew, spearmint, mustard, horseradish, lemon balm, sunflower, marigold, burdock, rosemary, mullein, borage, juniper

**Digestives**: Assists the stomach and intestines in normal digestion. Examples: caraway, spearmint, fennel, chamomile, horseradish, turmeric, ginger, yarrow, pineapple weed, chamomile, self-heal, sage, rosemary, juniper

**Diuretic**: Herbs that promote the secretion of urine. Examples: dandelion leaf, corn silk, parsley, cleavers, yarrow, parsley, carrot, sunflower, nettles, plantain, self-heal, burdock, mullein, goldenrod, juniper, rose hips

**Emetic**: Induces vomiting. Example: horseradish

**Emmenagogue**: Herb that brings on menstruation, and regulates, normalizes, and tones the female reproductive system. Examples: red raspberry, parsley, cinnamon, feverfew, marigold, juniper

**Emollient**: An application that softens, protects, and soothes the skin. Examples: plantain, chickweed, honey, avocado, mullein, borage

**Expectorant**: Herbs that help liquefy, loosen, and remove thick mucous from the lungs; quiets a cough and provides a tonic effect on the nervous system. Examples: mullein, thyme, watercress, fennel, parsley, caraway, garlic, onion, sunflower, plantain, burdock, red clover, heartsease, sweet violet, mullein, borage, rose hips

**Febrifuge**: Reduces body temperature and fever. Examples: yarrow, cayenne, garlic, ginger, cinnamon, ginger, chamomile, feverfew, spearmint, mustard, horseradish, lemon balm, sunflower, marigold, rosemary, borage

**Galactogogue**: Herbs that increase breast milk secretion in lactating moms. Examples: nettles, red raspberry, aniseed, caraway, fennel, carrot

**Hemostatic**: Astringent herbs that assist to stop bleeding. Examples: red raspberry, yarrow, cinnamon, cayenne, self-heal, nettle, plantain, sage

**Hepatic**: Promotes the tone, strength, and activity of the liver and increases the secretion of bile. Example: dandelion root, turmeric, marigold, yarrow

**Iatrogenic:** Of or relating to illness caused by medical examination or treatment, such as adverse effects, side effects, or medical errors.

**Laxative**: Herb that acts to promote evacuation of the bowels. Examples: dandelion root, chickweed, burdock, rose hips

**Lymphatic:** An agent that supports lymphatic drainage. Examples: red clover, nettles, cleavers, plantain, sweet violet

**Mucilaginous**: Herbs that soothe mucous membranes. Examples: plantain, corn silk

**Nervine**: Herbs that calm and soothe the nerves, reducing tension and anxiety. Examples: chamomile, lemon balm, Californian poppy, lavender, hops, pineapple weed, borage

**Ophthalmic:** A remedy for diseases of the eye. Example: carrot

**Parturifacient:** Herbs that induce labor; beneficial herbs during pregnancy. (**Parturient**) Example: red raspberry

**Poultice:** Powdered plants mixed with water to form a paste and applied to the skin to draw out infection and promote healing. Examples: plantain, chickweed, chamomile, self-heal, yarrow, marigold

**Refrigerant:** A cooling remedy that lowers body temperature. Examples: orange, lemon, chickweed, lemon balm, raspberry, cinnamon, rose

**Relaxant:** Relaxes and relieves tension, especially muscular tension (see sedative).

**Rubefacient:** An agent that causes an increase in surface blood flow, reddens the skin, and improves local circulation. Examples: cayenne, ginger, mustard, horseradish, thyme, juniper

**Sedative:** Herbs that calm down the nervous system, reduce excitement, and promote relaxation. Examples: lemon balm, chamomile, hops, lavender, California poppy, lavender, pineapple weed

**Stimulant:** A general term for an action that quickens, improves circulation, and increases the activity of an organ.

**Stomachic:** Herbs that give strength and tone to the stomach, stimulate digestion, and improve the appetite. Examples: ginger, turmeric, fennel

**Styptic:** Astringent—arrests hemorrhage and bleeding by contracting blood vessels and through blood coagulation. Examples: yarrow, plantain, cayenne, red raspberry, self-heal, marigold, sage

**Thymoleptic:** An herbal remedy that raises the mood and counteracts low spirits. Examples: lemon balm, feverfew, lavender

**Tincture**: A concentrated liquid solution that contains the soluble chemical constituents of plant roots, bark, seeds, and leaves.

**Tonic**: Herbs that restore, tone, and strengthen the entire body systems.

**Tonic (nutritive)**: An herb that has a normalizing effect on the body, working to regenerate cells and tissues and promoting strength and longevity. Example: red raspberry, nettles, red clover, burdock, chickweed

**Vermifuge** (anthelmintic, parasiticide, antiparasitic): An agent that expels intestinal worms or parasites. Examples: garlic, rosemary, cinnamon, turmeric, oregano, sage, feverfew, carrot, avocado, pineapple weed, oregano, marigold, carrot, thyme, rose hips

**Vulnerary**: An herb used to heal wounds and reduce inflammation, generally applied as a poultice. Example: honey, plantain, marigold, turmeric, chamomile, pineapple weed, chickweed, self-heal

# Resources

**Herbal Medicine References**
My personal website with loads of herbal medicine information and articles—www.katolenyardley.com

Alchemy & Elixir Health Group—www.alchemyelixir.com

National Institute of Medical Herbalists—www.nimh.org.uk

Canadian Herbalists Association of British Columbia—www.chaofbc.ca

Canadian Council of Herbalists Associations—www.herbalccha.org

American Herbalists Guild—www.americanherbalist.com

Richters Seeds—www.richters.com

United Plant Savers—www.unitedplantsavers.org

**Some of my favorite websites:**
Henriette's Herbal Homepage    http://www.henriettes-herb.com/
Monographs, herbal lore, photographs and a whole lot of the invaluable eclectic books freely accessible

Southwest School of Botanical Medicine    http://swsbm.com/ HOMEPAGE/HomePage.html
An invaluable website from the late Michael Moore - not the film maker but an herbalist. This website is full of fascinating plant lore, photos, lithographs, and reference manuals.

Lloyd Library    http://www.lloydlibrary.org/altmedresources.html
The largest pharmacognosy, botany and plant medicine library in the U.S.

The Herb Research Foundation    http://www.herbs.org/herbnews/
A nonprofit research & educational foundation focusing on worldwide use of herbs for health, environmental conservation & international development.

# ENDNOTES

1. Debasis Bagchi, Harry G. Preuss, and Anand Swaroop, eds., *Nutraceuticals and Functional Foods in Human Health and Disease Prevention* (Boca Raton, FL: CRC Press, Taylor & Francis Group, 2016), 667.
2. Ricardo Hernandez-Lambraño, Nerlis Pajaro-Castro, Karina Caballero-Gallardo, Elena Stashenko, and Jesus Olivero-Verbel. "Essential Oils from Plants of the Genus *Cymbopogon* as Natural Insecticides to Control Stored Product Pests," *Journal of Stored Products Research 62* (May 2015): 81–83, doi:10.1016/j.jspr.2015.04.004.
3. Edgar J. DaSilva, Elias Baydoun, and Adnan Badran, "Biotechnology and the Developing World," *Electronic Journal of Biotechnology* 5, no. 1 (2002), doi:10.2225/vol5-issue1-fulltext-1.
4. Interactive European Network for Industrial Crops and their Applications, *Summary Report for the European Union* (IENICA, 2005).
5. D. S. Fabricant and N. R. Farnsworth, "The Value of Plants Used in Traditional Medicine for Drug Discovery," *Environmental Health Perspec*tives 109 (March 2001): 69–75.
6. DaSilva, Baydoun, and Badran, "Biotechnology and the Developing World."
7. Word Health Organization, *WHO Traditional Medicine Strategy: 2014–2023* (Geneva: WHO Press, 2013), http://www.who.int/medicines/publications/traditional/trm_strategy14_23/en/.
8. "Pharmaceutical Industry," World Health Organization, http://www.who.int/trade/glossary/story073/en/.
9. "The Cost to End World Hunger," The Borgen Project, last modified Feb 15, 2013, http://borgenproject.org/the-cost-to-end-world-hunger/.
10. P. Rodríguez del Río, M. L. González-Gutiérrez, J. Sánchez-López, B. Nuñez-Acevedo, J. M. Bartolomé Álvarez, and C. Martínez-Cócera, "Urticaria Caused by Antihistamines: Report of 5 Cases," *Journal of Investigational Allergology and Clinical Immunology* 19, no. 4 (2009): 317–320.
11. H. Wolski, "Selected Aspects of Oral Contraception Side Effects," *Ginekologia Polska* 85, no. 12 (2014): 944–9.
12. Jennifer M. Gierisch, Remy R. Coeytaux, Rachel Peragallo Urrutia, Laura J. Havrilesky, Patricia G. Moorman, William J. Lowery, Michaela Dinan, Amanda J. McBroom, Vic Hasselblad, Gillian D. Sanders, and Evan R. Myers, "Oral Contraceptive Use and Risk of Breast, Cervical, Colorectal, and Endometrial Cancers: A Systematic Review," *Cancer Epidemiology, Biomarkers & Prevention, 22* (November 2013): 1931–43, doi: 10.1158/1055-9965.EPI-13-0298.
13. International Agency for Research on Cancer, "Combined Estrogen-Progestogen Contraceptives and Combined Estrogen-Progestogen Menopausal Therapy," *IARC Monographs on the Evaluation of Carcinogenic Risks to Humans* 91 (2007): 1–528.
14. Jayashri Kulkarni, "Depression as a Side Effect of the Contraceptive Pill," *Expert Opinion on Drug Safety* 6, no. 4 (July 2007): 371–4.

15. L. Poller, "Relation Between Oral Contraceptive Hormones and Blood Clotting," *Journal of Clinical Pathology Supplement* 3 (1969): 67–74.
16. A. Spinillo, E. Capuzzo, S. Nicola, F. Baltaro, A. Ferrari, A. Monaco, "The Impact of Oral Contraception on Vulvovaginal Candidiasis," *Contraception* 51, no. 5 (1995): 293–7.
17. J. D. Oriel, Betty M. Partridge, Maire J. Denny, J. C. Coleman, "Genital Yeast Infections," *British Medical Journal* 4 (1972): 761–764.
18. V. Moreno, F. X. Bosch, N. Muñoz, C. J. Meijer, K. V. Shah, J. M. Walboomers, R. Herrero, S. Franceschi, "Effect of Oral Contraceptives on Risk of Cervical Cancer in Women with Human Papillomavirus Infection: The IARC Multicentric Case-Control Study," *Lancet* 359 (March 2002): 1085–92.
19. Yogi Ramacharaka, *The Hindu-Yogi Science of Breath* (W. & J. Mackay & CG. Ltd., Chatham, UK, 1903), http://www.arfalpha.com/ScienceOfBreath/ScienceOfBreath.pdf.
20. Beverly Rubik, "The Biofield Hypothesis: Its Biophysical Basis and Role in Medicine," *The Journal of Alternative and Complementary Medicine* 8, no. 6 (July 2004): 703–717, doi:10.1089/10755530260511711.
21. A. R. Raji and R. E. Bowden, "Effects of High-Peak Pulsed Electromagnetic Field on the Degeneration and Regeneration of the Common Peroneal Nerve in Rats," *The Journal of Bone and Joint Surgery* 65, no. 4 (August 1983): 478–92.
22. J. M. Byers, K. F. Clark, and G. C. Thompson, "Effect of Pulsed Electromagnetic Stimulation on Facial Nerve Regeneration," *JAMA Otolaryngology—Head & Neck Surgery* 124, no. 4 (1998): 383–389, doi:10.1001/archotol.124.4.383.
23. S. L. Henry, M. J. Concannon, and G. J. Yee, "The Effect of Magnetic Fields on Wound Healing: Experimental Study and Review of the Literature," *Eplasty* 8 (July 2008).
24. C. Frank, N. Schachar, D. Dittrich, N. Shrive, W. deHaas, and G. Edwards, "Electromagnetic Stimulation of Ligament Healing in Rabbits," *Clinical Orthopaedics and Related Research* 175 (June 1983): 263–272.
25. G. Vighi, F. Marcucci, L. Sensi. G. Di Cara, and F. Frati, "Allergy and the Gastrointestinal System," *Clinical and Experimental Immunology* 153, no. 1 (2008): 3–6, doi: 10.1111/j.1365-2249.2008.03713.x.
26. K. Suzuki, S. A. Ha, M. Tsuji, and S. Fagarasan, "Intestinal IgA Synthesis: A Primitive Form of Adaptive Immunity That Regulates Microbial Communities in the Gut," *Seminars in Immunology* 19, no. 2 (2007): 127–35.
27. Katolen Yardley, *Introduction to Herbs for Holistic Nutritionists*. (Canadian School of Natural Nutrition. Advanced Nutrition Program. Ontario, Canada, 2011).
28. "Curcuma longa (Zingiberaceae)," J. A. Duke, *Dr. Duke's Phytochemical and Ethnobotanical Databases*, https://phytochem.nal.usda.gov/phytochem/plants/show/563?qlookup=+Curcuma+longa+L.+%E2%80%93+Zingiberaceae++&offset=0&-max=20&et=.
29. R. C. Wren, *Potter's New Cyclopaedia of Botanical Drugs and Preparations* (Essex, UK: The C. W. Daniel Company Limited, 1988).
30. Terry Willard, *Textbook of Modern Herbology* (Calgary: Progressive Publishing Inc., 1988).
31. Wren, *Potter's New Cyclopaedia*.
32. *USDA National Nutrient Database for Standard Reference Release 28: Full Report (All Nutrients) 11270, Mustard Greens, Raw*, report date: December 01, 2015.

33.  *USDA National Nutrient Database for Standard Reference Release 28: Basic Report 02024, Spices, Mustard Seed, Ground*, report date: December 01, 2015.

34.  Carol Newall, Linda Anderson, and David Phillipson, *Herbal Medicines: A Guide for Health-Care Professionals* (London: The Pharmaceutical Press, 1996).

35.  Sami Rokayya, Chun-Juan Li, Yan Zhao, Ying Li, and Chang-Hao Sun, "Cabbage (*Brassica oleracea* L. var. capitata) Phytochemicals with Antioxidant and Anti-inflammatory Potential," *Asian Pacific Journal of Cancer Prevention* 14 (2013): 6657–6662, doi: http://dx.doi.org/10.7314/APJCP.2013.14.11.6657.

36.  A. Vogel, *The Nature Doctor* (Teufen, Switzerland: Bioforce-Verlag, 1960), 18.

37.  A. Prawan, C. L. Saw, T. O. Khor, Y. S. Kheum, S. Yu, L. Hu, and A. N. Kong, "Anti-NF-kappaB and Anti-inflammatory Activities of Synthetic Isothiocyanates: Effect of Chemical Structures and Cellular Signaling," *Chemico-Biological Interactions* 179 (May 2009): 202–11.

38.  D. T. Verhoeven, R. A. Goldbohm, G. van Poppel, H. Verhagen, and P. A. van den Brandt, "Epidemiological Studies on Brassica Vegetables and Cancer Risk," *Cancer Epidemiology, Biomarkers & Prevention* 5 (1996):733–748.

39.  R. H. Liu, "Potential Synergy of Phytochemicals in Cancer Prevention: Mechanism of Action," *Journal of Nutrition* 134, no. 12 (December 2004): 3479S–3485S.

40.  J. L. Silberstein and J. K. Parsons, "Evidence-Based Principles of Bladder Cancer and Diet," *Urology* 75, no. 2 (February 2010): 340–6.

41.  M. A. Joseph, K. B. Moysich, J. L. Freudenheim, P. G. Shields, E. D. Bowman, Y. Zhang, J. R. Marshall, and C. B. Ambrosone, "Cruciferous Vegetables, Genetic Polymorphisms in Glutathione S-Transferases M1 and T1, and Prostate Cancer Risk," *Nutrition and Cancer* 50, no. 2 (2004): 206–13.

42.  Jane V. Higdon, Barbara Delage, David E. Williams, and Roderick H. Dashwood, "Cruciferous Vegetables and Human Cancer Risk: Epidemiologic Evidence and Mechanistic Basis," *Pharmacological Research* 55, no. 3 (2007): 224–236, doi: 10.1016/j.phrs.2007.01.009.

43.  Michael T. Murray, Joseph E. Pizzorno, and Lara Pizzorno, *The Encyclopedia of Healing Foods* (New York: Atria Books, 2005), 177.

44.  K. J. Auborn, S. Fan, E. M. Rosen, L. Goodwin, A. Chandraskaren, D. E. Williams, D. Chen, and T. H. Carter, "Indole-3-carbinol is a Negative Regulator of Estrogen," *Journal of Nutrition* 133 (July 2003): 2470S–2475S.

45.  R. Hu, T. O. Khor, G. Shen, W. S. Jeong, V. Hebbar, C. Chen, C. Xu, B. Reddy, K. Chada, and A. N. Kong, "Cancer Chemoprevention of Intestinal Polyposis in ApcMin/+ Mice by Sulforaphane, a Natural Product Derived from Cruciferous Vegetable," *Carcinogenesis* 27, no. 10 (May 2006): 2038–46.

46.  Vogel, *The Nature Doctor*, 193.

47.  B. Kusznierewicz, A. Bartoszek, L. Wolska. J. Drzewiecki, S. Gorinstein, and J. Namieśnik, "Partial Characterization of White Cabbages (*Brassica oleracea* var. capitata f. alba) from Different Regions by Glucosinolates, Bioactive Compounds, Total Antioxidant Activities, and Proteins," *LWT - Food Science and Technology* 41 (2008): 1–9.

48.  M. A. Greer, "Goitrogenic Substances in Food," *American Journal of Clinical Nutrition* 5, no. 4 (1957): 440–4.

49. M. S. Asadi, A. R. Mirvaghefei, M. A. Nematollahi, M. Banaee, and K. Ahmadi, "Effects of Watercress (*Nasturtium nasturtium*) Extract on Selected Immunological Parameters of Rainbow Trout (*Oncorhynchus mykiss*)," *Open Veterinary Journal* 2 (2012): 32–39.

50. *USDA National Nutrient Database for Standard Reference Release 28: Basic Report 11591, Watercress, Raw*, report date: November 30, 2015.

51. A. Seow, C. Y. Shi, F. L. Chung, D. Jiao, J. H. Hankin, H. P. Lee, G. A. Coetzee, and M. C. Yu, "Urinary Total isothiocyanate (ITC) in a Population-Based Sample of Middle-Aged and Older Chinese in Singapore: Relationship with Dietary Total ITC and Glutathione S-Transferase M1/T1/P1 Genotypes," *Cancer Epidemiology, Biomarkers & Prevention* 7 (September 1998): 775.

52. S. S. Hecht, S. G. Carmella, and S. E. Murphy, "Effects of Watercress Consumption on Urinary Metabolites of Nicotine in Smokers," *Cancer Epidemiology, Biomarkers & Prevention* 8, no. 10 (1999): 907–13.

53. Wen Tan, Nan Song, Gui-Qi Wang, Qing Liu, Huai-Jing Tang, Fred F. Kadlubar, and Dong-Xin Lin, "Impact of Genetic Polymorphisms in Cytochrome P450 2E1 and Glutathione S-Transferases M1, T1, and P1 on Susceptibility to Esophageal Cancer Among High-Risk Individuals in China," *Cancer Epidemiology, Biomarkers & Prevention* 9 (June 2000): 551.

54. S. S. Hecht, F. L. Chung, J. P. Richie Jr., S. A. Akerkar, A. Borukhova, L. Skowronski, and S. G. Carmella, "Effects of Watercress Consumption on Metabolism of a Tobacco-Specific Lung Carcinogen in Smokers," *Cancer Epidemiology, Biomarkers & Prevention* 4, no. 8 (December 1995): 877-84.

55. K. Liu, S. Cang, Y. Ma, and J. W. Chiao, "Synergistic Effect of Paclitaxel and Epigenetic Agent Phenethyl Isothiocyanate on Growth Inhibition, Cell Cycle Arrest and Apoptosis in Breast Cancer Cells," *Cancer Cell International* 13 (February 2013): 10, doi: 10.1186/1475-2867-13-10.

56. J. Croese, G. Chapman, and N. D. Gallagher, "Evolution of Fascioliasis After Eating Wild Watercress," *Australian and New Zealand Journal of Medicine* 12, no. 5 (October 1982): 525–7.

57. Wren, *Potter's New Cyclopaedia*.

58. *USDA National Nutrient Database for Standard Reference Release 28: Basic Report 02018, Spices, Fennel Seed*, report date: December 23, 2015.

59. "Polysorbate 80," TOXNET Toxicology Data Network, last modified October 15, 2010, http://toxnet.nlm.nih.gov/cgi-bin/sis/search/a?dbs+hsdb:@term+@DOCNO+4359

60. Benoit Chassaing, Omry Koren, Julia K. Goodrich, Angela C. Poole, Shanthi Srinivasan, Ruth E. Ley, and Andrew T. Gewirtz, "Dietary Emulsifiers Impact the Mouse Gut Microbiota Promoting Colitis and Metabolic Syndrome," *Nature* 519 (March 2015): 92–96, doi:10.1038/nature14232.

61. Carol L. Roberts, Åsa V. Keita, Sylvia H. Duncan, Niamh O'Kennedy, Johan D. Söderholm, Jonathan M. Rhodes, and Barry J. Campbell, "Translocation of Crohn's Disease *Escherichia coli* Across M-Cells: Contrasting Effects of Soluble Plant Fibres and Emulsifiers," *Gut* 59 (2010): 1331–9, doi:10.1136/gut.2009.195370.

62. Carol Newall, Linda Anderson, and David Phillipson, *Herbal Medicines: A Guide for Health-Care Professionals*, (London: The Pharmaceutical Press, 1996).

63. *USDA National Nutrient Database for Standard Reference Release 28: Basic Report 11124, Carrots, Raw*, report date: December 15, 2015.

64. "Carrot, Wild," M. Grieve, Botanical.com, https://www.botanical.com/botanical/mgm-h/c/carwil25.html.

65. Krishan Datt Sharma, Swati Karki, Narayan Singh Thakur, and Surekha Attri, "Chemical Composition, Functional Properties and Processing of Carrot—a Review," *Journal of Food Science and Technology* 49, no. 1 (February 2012): 22–32, doi: 10.1007/s13197-011-0310-7.

66. J. L. Silberstein and J. K. Parsons, "Evidence-Based Principles of Bladder Cancer and Diet," *Urology* 75, no. 2 (February 2010): 340–6. doi: 10.1016/j.urology.2009.07.1260.

67. R. Zaini, M. R. Clench, and C. L. Le Maitre, "Bioactive Chemicals from Carrot (Daucus carota) Juice Extracts for the Treatment of Leukemia," *Journal of Medicinal Food* 14, no. 11 (November 2011): 1303–12, doi: 10.1089/jmf.2010.0284.

68. M. Kobaek-Larsen, L. P. Christensen, W. Vach, J. Ritskes-Hoitinga, and K. Brandt, "Inhibitory Effects of Feeding with Carrots or (-)-Falcarinol on Development of Azoxymethane-Induced Preneoplastic Lesions in the Rat Colon," *Journal of Agricultural and Food Chemistry* 53, no. 5 (March 2005): 1823–7.

69. C. Zidorn, K. Jöhrer, M. Ganzera, B. Schubert, E. M. Sigmund, J. Mader, R. Greil, E. P. Ellmerer, and H. Stuppner, "Polyacetylenes from the Apiaceae Vegetables Carrot, Celery, Fennel, Parsley, and Parsnip and Their Cytotoxic Activities," *Journal of Agricultural and Food Chemistry* 53, no. 7 (April 2005): 2518–23.

70. A. Bishayee, A. Sarkar, and M. Chatterjee, "Hepatoprotective Activity of Carrot (Daucus carota L.) Against Carbon Tetrachloride Intoxication in Mouse Liver," *Journal of Ethnopharmacology* 47, no. 2 (July 1995): 69–74.

71. Newall, Anderson, and Phillipson, *Herbal Medicines*.

72. "How to Identify Queen Anne's Lace (Wild Carrot)," Leah Lefler, HubPages, last modified on June 18, 2012, http://hubpages.com/living/How-to-Identify-Queen-Annes-Lace-Wild-Carrot

73. Wren, *Potter's New Cyclopaedia*.

74. *USDA National Nutrient Database for Standard Reference Release 28: Basic Report 11297, Parsley, Fresh*, report date: December 15, 2015.

75. Chanchal Cabrera, *Fibromyalgia: A Journey Toward Healing* (New York: Contemporary Books, 2002), 286.

76. Ibid.

77. Wren, *Potter's New Cyclopaedia*.

78. Eva Nemeth, ed., *Caraway: The Genus Carum* (Amsterdam: Harwood Academic Publishers, 1998), 39

79. *USDA National Nutrient Database for Standard Reference Release 28: Basic Report 02005, Spices, Caraway Seed*, report date: December 23, 2015.

80. Willard, *Textbook of Modern Herbology*, 274.

81. Wren, *Potter's New Cyclopaedia*.

82. Ibid.

83. Newall, Anderson, and Phillipson, *Herbal Medicines*.

84. Newall, Anderson, and Phillipson, *Herbal Medicines*.

85. Wren, *Potter's New Cyclopaedia*.

86. *USDA National Nutrient Database for Standard Reference Release 28: Basic Report 11282, Onions, Raw*, report date: December 23, 2015.

87. B. Chempakam and V. A. Parthasarathy, "Turmeric," in *Chemistry of Spices*, ed. V. A. Parthasarathy, B. Chempakam, and T. J. Zachariah (Cambridge, MA: CABI Publishing, 2008), 97.

88. Sahdeo Prasad and Bharat B. Aggarwal, "Turmeric, the Golden Spice: From Traditional Medicine to Modern Medicine," in *Herbal Medicine: Biomolecular and Clinical Aspects, 2nd edition*, ed. I. F. F. Benzie and S. Wachtel-Galor (Boca Raton, FL: CRC Press/Taylor & Francis, 2011).

89. Wren, *Potter's New Cyclopaedia*.

90. B. B. Aggarwal, W. Yuan, S. Li, and S. C. Gupta, "Curcumin-Free Turmeric Exhibits Anti-inflammatory and Anticancer Activities: Identification of Novel Components of Turmeric," *Molecular Nutrition & Food Research* 57, no. 9 (September 2013): 1529–42, doi: 10.1002/mnfr.201200838.

91. B. White and D. Z. Judkins, "Does Turmeric Relieve Inflammatory Conditions?" *Journal of Family Practice* 60, no. 3 (March 2011), 155–156.

92. S. D. Deodhar, R. Sethi, and R. C. Srimal, "Preliminary Studies on Antirheumatic Activity of Curcumin (Diferuloyl Methane)," *Indian Journal of Medical Research* 71 (April 1980): 632–634.

93. Kerry Bone and Simon Mills, *Principles and Practice of Phytotherapy: Modern Herbal Medicine* (London: Harcourt Publishers Limited, 2000).

94. S. K. Kurd, N. Smith, A. VanVoorhees, A. B. Troxel, V. Badmaev, J. T. Seykora, and J. M. Gelfand, "Oral Curcumin in the Treatment of Moderate to Severe Psoriasis Vulgaris: A Prospective Clinical Trial," *Journal of the American Academy of Dermatology* 58, no. 4 (April 2008): 625–631.

95. M. C. Heng, M. K. Song, J. Harker, M. K. Heng, "Drug-Induced Suppression of Phosphorylase Kinase Activity Correlates with Resolution of Psoriasis as Assessed by Clinical, Histological, and Immunohistochemical Parameters, *British Journal of Dermatology* 143, no. 5 (November 2000): 937–949.

96. S. U. *Zaman and N. Akhtar*, "Effect of Turmeric (Curcuma longa Zingiberaceae) Extract Cream on Human Skin Sebum Secretion," *Tropical Journal of Pharmaceutical Research* 12, no. 5 (October 2013): 665–669.

97. F. Zhang, N. K. Altorki, J. R. Mestre, K. Subbaramaiah, A. J. Dannenberg, "Curcumin Inhibits Cyclooxygenase-2 Transcription in Bile Acid- and Phorbol Ester-Treated Human Gastrointestinal Epithelial Cells," *Carcinogenesis* 20, no. 3 (March 1999): 445–51.

98. Bone and Mills, *Principles and Practice of Phytotherapy*.

99. S. M. Sagar, D. Yance, and R. K. Wong, "Natural Health Products that Inhibit Angiogenesis: A Potential Source for Investigational New Agents to Treat Cancer—Part 1," *Current Oncology* 13, no. 1 (February 2006): 14–26.

100. Y. Aratanechemuge, T. Komiya, H. Moteki, H. Katsuzaki, K. Imai, and H. Hibasami, "Selective Induction of Apoptosis by Ar-Turmerone Isolated from Turmeric (Curcuma longa L.) in Two Human Leukemia Cell Lines, but Not in Human Stomach Cancer Cell Line," *International Journal of Molecular Medicine* 9, no. 5 (2002): 481–4.

101. Ekram M. Saleh, Raafat A El-awady, Nadia A. Eissa, and Wael M. Abdel-Rahman, "Antagonism Between Curcumin and the Topoisomerase II Inhibitor Etoposide: A Study of DNA Damage, Cell Cycle Regulation and Death Pathways," *Cancer Biology & Therapy* 13, no. 11 (September 2012): 1058–1071, doi: 10.4161/cbt.21078.

102. P. R. Holt, S. Katz, and R. Kirshoff, "Curcumin Therapy in Inflammatory Bowel Disease: A Pilot Study," *Digestive Diseases and Sciences* 50, no. 11 (November 2005): 2191–3.

103. H. Hanai, T. Iida, K. Takeuchi, F. Watanabe, Y. Maruyama, A. Andoh, T. Tsujikawa, et al., "Curcumin Maintenance Therapy for Ulcerative Colitis: Randomized, Multicenter, Double-Blind, Placebo-Controlled Trial," *Clinical Gastroenterology and Hepatology* 4, no. 12 (December 2006): 1502–1506.

104. T. Kawamori, R. Lubet, V. E. Steele, G. J. Kelloff, R. B. Kaskey, C. V. Rao, B. S. Reddy, "Chemopreventive Effect of Curcumin, a Naturally Occurring Anti-inflammatory Agent, During the Promotion/Progression Stages of Colon Cancer," *Cancer Research* 59 (February 1999): 597–601.

105. Cabrera, *Fibromyalgia*, 259.

106. Chhavi Sharma, Pooja Suhalka, Piyu Sukhwal, Neha Jaiswal, and Maheep Bhatnagar, "Curcumin Attenuates Neurotoxicity Induced by Fluoride: An *in vivo* Evidence," *Pharmacognosy Magazine* 10, no. 37 (2014): 61–65, doi: 10.4103/0973-1296.126663.

107. "Sources of Flouride," Fluoride Action Network, http://fluoridealert.org/issues/sources/.

108. Bone and Mills, *Principles and Practice of Phytotherapy*.

109. Ibid.

110. Wren, *Potter's New Cyclopaedia*.

111. Newall, Anderson, and Phillipson, *Herbal Medicines*.

112. Ibid.

113. Aviva Jill Romm, *The Natural Pregnancy Book: Herbs, Nutrition, and Other Holistic Choices* (Berkley, CA: Celestial Arts, 2003).

114. Wren, *Potter's New Cyclopaedia*.

115. Newall, Anderson, and Phillipson, *Herbal Medicines*.

116. *USDA National Nutrient Database for Standard Reference Release 28: Basic Report 02031, Spices, Pepper, Red or Cayenne*, report date: December 26, 2015.

117. Newall, Anderson, and Phillipson, *Herbal Medicines*.

118. "Nonsteroidal Anti-inflammatory Drug," *Wikipedia*, accessed December 12, 2015, https://en.wikipedia.org/wiki/Nonsteroidal_anti-inflammatory_drug.

119. G. Singh, "Recent Considerations in Nonsteroidal Anti–inflammatory Drug Gastropathy," *American Journal of Medicine* 105 (July 1998): 31S–38S.

120. "Bayer Annual Report, 2013, Table 3.15.3," Bayer, last modified February 28, 2014, http://www.annualreport2013.bayer.com/en/healthcare.aspx.

121. "Bayer Annual Report, 2013, Table 3.15.5," Bayer, last modified February 28, 2014, http://www.annualreport2013.bayer.com/en/healthcare.aspx.

122. M. Yasir, S. Das, and M. D. Kharya. "The Phytochemical and Pharmacological Profile of *Persea americana* Mill," *Pharmacognosy Reviews* 4, no. 7 (2010): 77–84, doi: 10.4103/0973-7847.65332.

123. Mark L. Dreher and Adrienne J. Davenport, "Hass Avocado Composition and Potential Health Effects," *Critical Reviews in Food Science and Nutrition* 53, no. 7 (2013): 738–750, doi: 10.1080/10408398.2011.556759.

124. Ibid.

125. "Monograph: Avocado and Garlic," Luke Robinson, http://www.academia.edu/7913968/Monograph_Avocado_and_Garlic.

126. N. Z. Unlu, T. Bohn, S. K. Clinton, and S. J. Schwartz, "Carotenoid Absorption from Salad and Salsa by Humans is Enhanced by the Addition of Avocado or Avocado Oil," *Journal of Nutrition* 135, no. 3 (March 2005): 431–6.

127. Mark L. Dreher and Adrienne J. Davenport, "Hass Avocado Composition and Potential Health Effects," *Critical Reviews in Food Science and Nutrition* 53, no. 7 (2013): 738–750, doi: 10.1080/10408398.2011.556759.

128. Z. Pieterse, J. C. Jerling, W. Oosthuizen, H. S. Kruger, S. M. Hanekom, C. M. Smuts, and A. E. Schutte, "Substitution of High Monounsaturated Fatty Acid Avocado for Mixed Dietary Fats During an Energy-Restricted Diet: Effects on Weight Loss, Serum Lipids, Fibrinogen, and Vascular Function," *Nutrition* 21, no. 1 (January 2005): 67–75.

129. W. C. Grant, "Influence of Avocados on Serum Cholesterol," *Proceedings of the Society for Experimental Biology and Medicine*, 104 (May 1960): 45–7.

130. J. Carranza, M. Alvizouri, M. R. Alvarado, F. Chávez, M. Gómez, and J. E. Herrera, "Effects of Avocado on the Level of Blood Lipids in Patients with Phenotype II and IV Dyslipidemias," *Archivos del Instituto Cardiología de México* 65, no. 4 (1995): 342–8.

131. M. Yasir, S. Das, and M. D. Kharya. "The Phytochemical and Pharmacological Profile of *Persea americana* Mill," *Pharmacognosy Reviews* 4, no. 7 (2010): 77–84, doi: 10.4103/0973-7847.65332.

132. Wren, *Potter's New Cyclopaedia.*

133. Newall, Anderson, and Phillipson, *Herbal Medicines.*

134. Wren, *Potter's New Cyclopaedia.*

135. Ibid.

136. Newall, Anderson, and Phillipson, *Herbal Medicines.*

137. Bone and Mills, *Principles and Practice of Phytotherapy.*

138. Newall, Anderson, and Phillipson, *Herbal Medicines.*

139. Bone and Mills, *Principles and Practice of Phytotherapy.*

140. Ibid.

141. Ibid.

142. Wren, *Potter's New Cyclopaedia.*

143. Donald Yance, *Herbal Medicine, Healing & Cancer: A Comprehensive Program for Prevention and Treatment* (Chicago: Keats Publishing, 1999), 143.

144. Wren, *Potter's New Cyclopaedia.*

145. Cabrera, *Fibromyalgia*, 278.

146. Ibid.

147. Wren, *Potter's New Cyclopaedia.*

148. Newall, Anderson, and Phillipson, *Herbal Medicines.*

149. Ibid.

150. Wren, *Potter's New Cyclopaedia.*

151. Gazmend Skenderi, *Herbal Vade Mecum* (Rutherford, NJ: Herbacy Press, 2003), 221.

152. Timothy F. Loomis, Chaomei Ma, and Mohsen Daneshtalab, "Medicinal Plants and Herbs of Newfoundland. Part 1. Chemical Constituents of the Aerial Part of Pineapple Weed (*Matricaria matricarioides*)," *DARU Journal of Pharmaceutical Sciences* 12, no. 4 (2004): 131–135.

153. The European Agency for the Evaluation of Medicinal Products Veterinary Medicines Evaluation Unit, *Committee for Veterinary Medicinal Products: Bellis Perennis Summary Report* (August 1999), http://www.ema.europa.eu/docs/en_GB/document_library/ Maximum_Residue_Limits_-_Report/2009/11/WC500010965.pdf.

154. "A New Look at Daisy (Bellis Perennis)," Anne McIntyre, *Positive Health Online*, modified June 2012, http://www.positivehealth.com/article/ herbal-medicine/a-new-look-at-daisy-bellis-perennis.

155. Wren, *Potter's New Cyclopaedia.*

156. *USDA National Nutrient Database for Standard Reference Release 28: Basic Report 12036, Seeds, Sunflower Seed Kernels, Dried*, report date: December 24, 2015.

157. "Sunflower," M. Grieve, Botanical.com, https://www.botanical.com/botanical/mgm-h/s/sunfl100.html.

158. *USDA National Nutrient Database for Standard Reference Release 28: Basic Report 12036, Seeds, Sunflower Seed Kernels, Dried*, report date: December 24, 2015.

159. Wren, *Potter's New Cyclopaedia.*

160. Newall, Anderson, and Phillipson, *Herbal Medicines.*

161. Ibid.

162. Wren, *Potter's New Cyclopaedia.*

163. Steve Brill, *Shoots and Greens of Early Spring in Northeastern North America* (New York: "Wildman" Steve Brill, 2008).

164. Willard, *Textbook of Modern Herbology*, 204.

165. Wren, *Potter's New Cyclopaedia.*

166. Newall, Anderson, and Phillipson, *Herbal Medicines.*

167. Skenderi, *Herbal Vade Mecum*, 300.

168. Newall, Anderson, and Phillipson, *Herbal Medicines.*

169. Wren, *Potter's New Cyclopaedia.*

170. Newall, Anderson, and Phillipson, *Herbal Medicines.*

171. *USDA National Nutrient Database for Standard Reference Release 28: Basic Report 11207, Dandelion Greens, Raw*, report date: December 24, 2015.

172. "Prunella vulgaris: Self-Heal," Anne Mcintyre, http://annemcintyre.com/ prunella-vulgaris-self-heal/.

173. Wren, *Potter's New Cyclopaedia.*

174. "Prunella vulgaris: Self-Heal," Anne Mcintyre, http://annemcintyre.com/ prunella-vulgaris-self-heal/.

175. S. Foster and R. Johnson, *Desk Reference to Nature's Medicine* (Washington, DC: National Geographic Society, 2006).

176. J. L. Lamaison, C. Petitjean-Freytet, and A. Carnat, "Medicinal Lamiaceae with Antioxidant Properties, a Potential Source of Rosmarinic Acid," *Pharmaceutica Acta Helvetiae* 66, no. 7 (1991): 185–8.

177. H. Markova, J. Sousek, and J. Ulrichova, "Prunella vulgaris L.–A Rediscovered Medicinal Plant," *Ceska Slov Farm* 46, no. 2 (April 1997): 58–63.

178. H. Lee and J. Y. Lin, "Antimutagenic Activity of Extracts from Anticancer Drugs in Chinese Medicine," *Mutation Research* 204, no. 2 (February 1998): 229–34.

179. Skenderi, *Herbal Vade Mecum*, 304.

180. Wren, *Potter's New Cyclopaedia.*

181. Newall, Anderson, and Phillipson, *Herbal Medicines*.
182. Yinrong Lu and L. Yeap Foo, "Antioxidant Activities of Polyphenols from Sage (*Salvia officinalis*)," *Food Chemistry* 75, no. 2 (November 2001): 197–202.
183. David O. Kennedy, Sonia Pace, Crystal Haskell, Edward J. Okello, Anthea Milne, and Andrew B. Scholey, "Effects of Cholinesterase Inhibiting Sage (*Salvia officinalis*) on Mood, Anxiety and Performance on a Psychological Stressor Battery," *Neuropsychopharmacology* 31, no. 4 (April 2006): 845–852, doi:10.1038/sj.npp.1300907.
184. Maryam Eidi, Akram Eidi, and Massih Bahar, "Effects of *Salvia officinalis* L. (Sage) Leaves on Memory Retention and Its Interaction with the Cholinergic System in Rats," *Nutrition* 22, no. 3 (March 2006): 321–326.
185. Teresa Iuvone, Daniele De Filippis, Giuseppe Esposito, Alessandra D'Amico, and Angelo A. Izzo, "The Spice Sage and Its Active Ingredient Rosmarinic Acid Protect PC12 Cells from Amyloid-β Peptide-Induced Neurotoxicity," *Journal of Pharmacology and Experimental Therapeutics* 317, no. 3 (June 2006): 1143–9, doi:10.1124/jpet.105.099317.
186. S. Bommer, P. Klein, and A. Suter, "First Time Proof of Sage's Tolerability and Efficacy in Menopausal Women with Hot Flushes," *Advances in Therapy* 28, no. 6 (June 2011): 490–500, doi: 10.1007/s12325-011-0027-z.
187. A. Mohagheghzadeh, P. Faridi, M. Shams-Ardakani, and Y. Ghasemi, "Medicinal Smokes," *Journal of Ethnopharmacology* 108, no. 2 (November 2006): 161–84.
188. Wren, *Potter's New Cyclopaedia*.
189. Newall, Anderson, and Phillipson, *Herbal Medicines*.
190. *USDA National Nutrient Database for Standard Reference Release 28: Full Report (All Nutrients) 11105, Burdock Root, Cooked, Boiled, Drained, Without Salt*, report date: December 24, 2015.
191. Amanda McQuade Crawford, *The Natural Menopause Handbook: Herbs, Nutrition, and Other Natural Therapies* (New York: Crossing Press, 2009), 100.
192. Wren, *Potter's New Cyclopaedia*.
193. Newall, Anderson, and Phillipson, *Herbal Medicines*.
194. "How to Tell the Difference Between Violas and Pansies," Deborah Stone, *Sunday Express*, last modified Feb 12, 2015, http://www.express.co.uk/life-style/garden/557646/How-tell-difference-between-violas-pansies.
195. Francis Edward Stewart, *A Compend of Pharmacy: Based Upon J. R. Remington's "Text-Book of Pharmacy"* (Philadelphia: P. Blakinston, Son & Co., 1886), 178.
196. Wren, *Potter's New Cyclopaedia*.
197. Skenderi, *Herbal Vade Mecum*, 187.
198. Wren, *Potter's New Cyclopaedia*.
199. S. L. Gerlach, R. Rathinakumar, G. Chakravarty, U. Göransson, W. C. Wimley, S. P. Darwin, and D. Mondal, "Anticancer and Chemosensitizing Abilities of Cycloviolacin O2 from Viola odorata and Psyle Cylotides from Psychotria leptothyrsa," *Biopolymers* 94, no. 5 (2010): 617–25.
200. M. A. Ebrahimzadeh, S. M. Nabavi, S. F. Nabavi, F. Bahramian, and A. R. Bekhradnia, "Antioxidant and Free Radical Scavenging Activity of H. Officinalis L. Var. Angustifolius, V. Odorata, B. Hyrcana and C. Speciosum," *Pakistan Journal of Pharmaceutical Sciences* 23, no. 1 (January 2010): 29–34.

201. "Bedstraw, Lady's," M. Grieve, Botanical.com, https://www.botanical.com/botanical/mgmh/b/bedlad25.html.

202. Wren, *Potter's New Cyclopaedia*.

203. Ibid.

204. Newall, Anderson, and Phillipson, *Herbal Medicines*.

205. David Winston and Steven Maimes, *Adaptogens: Herbs for Strength, Stamina, and Stress Relief* (Rochester, VT: Healing Arts Press, 2007).

206. Melody M. Bomgardner, "Food Additives: Extending Shelf Life with Natural Preservatives," *Chemical & Engineering News* 92, no. 6 (February 2014): 13–14.

207. Wren, *Potter's New Cyclopaedia*.

208. Nazia Masood Ahmed Chaudhry, Sabahat Saeed, and Perween Tariq, "Antibacterial Effects of Oregano (*Origanum Vulgare*) Against Gram Negative Bacilli," *Pakistan Journal of Botany* 39, no. 2 (2007): 609–613.

209. Skenderi, *Herbal Vade Mecum*, 372.

210. Newall, Anderson, and Phillipson, *Herbal Medicines*.

211. Ruth Trickey, *Women, Hormones & The Menstrual Cycle*, (Australia: Allen & Unwin, 1998), 320–321, 1998.

212. Trickey, *Women, Hormones & The Menstrual Cycle*, 322.

213. *USDA National Nutrient Database for Standard Reference Release Full Report (All Nutrients): 09302, Raspberries, Raw.*

214. Katolen Yardley, "Introduction to Herbs for Holistic Nutritionists" (workbook, Canadian School of Natural Nutrition Advanced Nutrition Program, Ontario, Canada, 2011).

215. Cabrera, *Fibromyalgia*, 248.

216. Wren, *Potter's New Cyclopaedia*.

217. Newall, Anderson, and Phillipson, *Herbal Medicines*.

218. W. F. Erdmann, "Phytoncides. I. Lupulone and Humulone; Their Antibacterial Action and Their Use in Tuberculous Infections," *Die Pharmazie* 6, no. 9 (September 1951): 442–51.

219. J. C. Lewis, G. Alderton, J. F. Carson. D. M. Reynolds, and W. D. MacLay, "Lupulon and Humulon-Antibiotic Constituents of Hops," *Journal of Clinical Investigation* 28 (September 1949): 916–9, doi:10.1172/JCI102178.

220. Wren, *Potter's New Cyclopaedia*.

221. McQuade Crawford, *The Natural Menopause Handbook*, 100.

222. S. R. Milligan, J. C. Kalita, A. Heyerick, H. Rong, L. De Cooman, and D. De Keukeleire, "Identification of a Potent Phytoestrogen in Hops (Humulus lupulus L.) and Beer," *Journal of Clinical Endocrinology and Metabolism* 84, no. 6 (June 1999): 2249–52.

223. Theresa L. Crenshaw and James P. Goldberg, *Sexual Pharmacology: Drugs that Affect Sexual Function* (New York: W. W. Norton and Co., 1996).

224. McQuade Crawford, *The Natural Menopause Handbook*, 101.

225. H. Adlercreutz, "Phyto-Oestrogens and Cancer," *The Lancet Oncology* 3, no. 6 (June 2002): 364–73, doi:10.1016/S1470-2045(02)00777-5.

226. P. Sunita and S. P. Pattanayak, "Phytoestrogens in Postmenopausal Indications: A Theoretical Perspective," *Pharmacognosy Reviews* 5, no. 9 (2011): 41–47, doi: 10.4103/0973-7847.79098.

227. H. R. Lindner, "Occurrence of Anabolic Agents in Plants and Their Importance," *Environmental Quality and Safety Supplement* 5 (*1976*): 151–8.
228. Cabrera, *Fibromyalgia*, 271.
229. Bone and Mills, *Principles and Practice of Phytotherapy*.
230. Wren, *Potter's New Cyclopaedia*.
231. Newall, Anderson, and Phillipson, *Herbal Medicines*.
232. Cabrera, *Fibromyalgia*, 301.
233. *USDA National Nutrient Database for Standard Reference Release 28: Basic Report 35205, Stinging Nettles, Blanched (Northern Plains Indians)*, report date: December 24, 2015.
234. Bone and Mills, *Principles and Practice of Phytotherapy*.
235. Wren, *Potter's New Cyclopaedia*.
236. Newall, Anderson, and Phillipson, *Herbal Medicines*.
237. Katolen Yardley, *Introduction to Herbs for Holistic Nutritionists.* (Canadian School of Natural Nutrition. Advanced Nutrition Program. Ontario, Canada, 2011).
238. Willard, *Textbook of Modern Herbology*, 201.
239. Wren, *Potter's New Cyclopaedia*.
240. Skenderi, *Herbal Vade Mecum*, 259.
241. Wren, *Potter's New Cyclopaedia*.
242. R. F. Weiss, *Herbal Medicine* (Beaconsfield, England: Beaconsfield Publishers, 1988), 241-242.
243. Beverly Gray, *The Boreal Herbal: Wild Food and Medicine Plants of the North* (Yukon, Canada: Aroma Borealis Press, 2011), 100.
244. Wren, *Potter's New Cyclopaedia*.
245. Skenderi, *Herbal Vade Mecum*, 321.
246. *USDA National Nutrient Database for Standard Reference Release 28: Basic Report 35203, Rose Hips, Wild (Northern Plains Indians)*, report date: December 22, 2015.
247. *USDA National Nutrient Database for Standard Reference Release 28: Basic Report 09202, Oranges, Raw, Navels*, report date: December 22, 2015.
248. R. Jenkins, N. Burton, and R. Cooper, "Manuka Honey Inhibits Cell Division in Methicillin-Resistant Staphylococcus aureus," *Journal of Antimicrobial Chemotherapy* 66, no. 11 (November 2011): 2536–42, doi: 10.1093/jac/dkr340.
249. P. H. Kwakman, A. A. te Velde, L. de Boer, D. Speijer, C. M. Vandenbroucke-Grauls, and S. A. Zaat, "How Honey Kills Bacteria," *FASEB Journal* 24, no. 7 (July 2010): 2576–82, doi: 10.1096/fj.09-150789.
250. Ibid.
251. R. J. Weston, "The Contribution of Catalase and Other Natural Products to the Antibacterial Activity of Honey: A Review," *Food Chemistry* 71, no. 2 (2000): 235–239.
252. World Health Organization, *Cough and Cold Remedies for the Treatment of Acute Respiratory Infections in Young Children* (Geneva: World Health Organization, 2001).
253. "New Study Finds Major Toxins in Many Cosmetics," J. M. Mercola, Mercola.com, last modified June 04, 2011, http://articles.mercola.com/sites/articles/archive/2011/06/04/new-study-finds-major-toxins-in-many-cosmetics.aspx.

# INDEX